DERMATOLOGICAL
SURGERY

Other titles forthcoming in the *New Clinical Applications* Series:

Dermatology (Series Editor Dr J. Verbov)
Talking Points in Dermatology
Superficial Fungal Infections
Treatment in Dermatology

Cardiology (Series Editor Dr D. Longmore)
Cardiology Screening

Gastroenterology (Series Editor Prof. S. Matern)

Rheumatology (Series Editors Dr J. J. Calabro and Dr W. Carson Dick)

NEW
CLINICAL
APPLICATIONS
DERMATOLOGY

DERMATOLOGICAL SURGERY

Editor

JULIAN L. VERBOV

JP, MD, FRCP, FIBiol

Consultant Dermatologist
Royal Liverpool Hospital,
Liverpool, UK

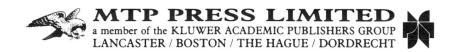

MTP PRESS LIMITED
a member of the KLUWER ACADEMIC PUBLISHERS GROUP
LANCASTER / BOSTON / THE HAGUE / DORDRECHT

Published in the UK and Europe by
MTP Press Limited
Falcon House
Lancaster, England

British Library Cataloguing in Publication Data

Dermatological surgery.—(New clinical applications.
  Dermatology)
  1. Skin—Surgery
  I. Verbov, Julian   II. Series
  617'.477   RD520

  ISBN 0-85200-934-8
  ISBN 0-85200-823-6 series

Published in the USA by
MTP Press
A division of Kluwer Boston Inc
190 Old Derby Street
Hingham, MA 02043, USA

Typeset and printed by Butler & Tanner Ltd,
Frome and London

CONTENTS

LIST OF AUTHORS

Mr J. A. S. Carruth, FRCS
Consultant Otolaryngologist
Royal South Hants Hospital
Graham Road
Southampton
SO9 4PE

Dr J. S. Comaish, MD, FRCP
Consultant Dermatologist
The Royal Victoria Infirmary
Queen Victoria Road
Newcastle upon Tyne
NE1 4LP

Dr R. P. R. Dawber, MA, FRCP
Consultant Dermatologist
The Slade Hospital
Headington
Oxford
OX3 7JH

Prof. E. Haneke, MD
Department of Dermatology
University of Erlangen-Nürnberg
Hartmannstr. 14
D-8520 Erlangen
FRG

SERIES EDITOR'S FOREWORD

This is the first volume of a series of regularly appearing books providing an authoritative update on selected topics in dermatology. *Dermatological Surgery* is a most appropriate volume to begin the series being an example of a rapidly expanding specialty within dermatology.

The four contributing authors are at the forefront of this exciting subject and they each have written a stimulating and informative chapter.

I hope that dermatologists, dermatologists in training, all those with an interest in skin disease, and there are many, and our friends specializing in plastic surgery, will all derive much benefit from the book.

JULIAN VERBOV

ABOUT THE EDITOR

Dr Julian Verbov is Consultant Dermatologist to Liverpool Health Authority and Clinical Lecturer in Dermatology at the University of Liverpool.

He is a member of the British Association of Dermatologists representing the British Society for Paediatric Dermatology on its Executive Committee. He is a Council Member of the Dermatology Section of the Royal Society of Medicine, and a Committee Member of the North of England Dermatological Society.

He is a fellow of the Institute of Biology and of the Zoological Society of London and a Member of the Society of Authors. He is a popular speaker and author of some 175 publications. His special interests include paediatric dermatology, inherited disorders, dermatoglyphics, pruritus ani, therapeutics, and medical humour. He organizes the British Postgraduate Course in Paediatric Dermatology and is a Member of the Editorial Boards of both *Clinical and Experimental Dermatology* and *Pediatric Dermatology*.

1
DERMATOLOGICAL SURGERY

J. S. COMAISH

HISTORY AND TRADITION

The recent history of dermatology in this country is that of a medical not a surgical speciality, as witnessed by the all-important role and status attached to the MRCP examination. The foundations of the speciality, however, were as firmly laid by surgeons as by physicians – the names of Paget, Jonathan Hutchinson, and Erasmus Wilson spring to mind. That dermatology developed along medical rather than surgical lines seems almost an accident of history; it could so easily have gone the opposite way. Recently the early roots of dermatology have been re-traced and the concept of this discipline as an organ speciality, embodying both medical and surgical skills for its practice, has been promulgated. There is much to commend this unified approach, as has been discovered in the sister specialities of ophthalmology and otorhinolaryngology. A unified approach also seems best for the patient, who is spared the expense and trouble of cross-referrals. For a health service whose watchwords are efficiency and economy this approach should have appeal; and for the practitioner there is more complete fulfilment in practising with all the skills available to him, some of which may have lain dormant since his house surgeon days.

The development of dermatology as a surgical speciality also confers distinct benefits on plastic surgeons, whose enormous waiting lists can be purged of the humdrum moles, tattoos, rodent ulcers and so on, which clog their busy schedule, leaving them more time to devote to developing special interests in microvascular surgery, joint prostheses and major reconstructions using myocutaneous flaps and so on.

For some plastic surgeons this blessing is too well disguised to acclaim, but I feel the climate of opinion is gradually changing and the advantage of cooperation, as for example in Mohs' surgery, will become steadily clearer.

CHANGE

Change is inevitable if not always welcomed. Dermatology has always had a strong surgical component in Europe (especially Germany) and the USA. The shift in emphasis of the last decade has come about for a number of reasons. The stimulus in some ways is evident – the growth of family and community medicine in the USA and elsewhere has produced a new and enterprising breed of physicians willing and able to practise dermatology to a competent if not specialist standard in their own milieu. They have forced dermatologists to look to their laurels – and their bank balances – with a keener eye. Encouragement has also come from the patients themselves, and their insurers – the diagnosis and treatment of the common skin tumours and cosmetic blemishes usually come cheaper and quicker than by being referred for plastic surgery.

A number of original-minded dermatologists have produced genuine advances in the field – Orentreich's work on hair transplant surgery opened a new era in cosmetic surgery; Shelley's detailed laboratory work on axillary hyperhidrosis led to a new successful and simple surgical technique for dealing with this troublesome condition. The *Journal of Dermatological Surgery and Oncology* is full of interesting 'jewels' or original articles of no outstanding scientific worth, but often indicating great experience and originality. The accumulation and dissemination of this type of knowledge is gradually changing the whole practice of dermatology.

PRESENT STATUS OF DERMATOLOGICAL SURGERY

World-wide it cannot be doubted that, in this as in many other fields, the energy and enterprise of the USA have been predominant. In most centres there we see sub-departments and departments of dermatological surgery flourishing or being established. In these places a great range of procedures is undertaken – from simple tumour excision to Mohs' surgery with flap and graft repairs; from cryosurgery to dermabrasion.

In many centres a good working relationship has been established with plastic surgeons, ENT and ophthalmic surgeons. The International Society for Dermatologic Surgery has done much to foster such good relations and many articles in its official journal (the *Journal of Dermatologic Surgery and Oncology*) are by surgeons. The ISDS Annual Meeting of 1984 in Jerusalem was organized locally by a plastic surgeon, and many of the contributions both in discussion and by papers were by plastic surgeons. This interplay of specialized areas of knowledge bodes well for the future. In the United Kingdom work along these lines only became formalized in 1982 when a group of dermatologists from Newcastle, Oxford and Plymouth founded the British Dermatological Surgery Group, which became affiliated to the British Association of Dermatologists the following year. That the time was ripe for this development is indicated by the fact that not a single dissenting voice was raised against the establishment of this group. Since 1982 two practical workshops have been organized in Newcastle; another is planned for 1986 in Plymouth, and another for 1987 in Oxford. Their aim is to teach young dermatologists how to do simple procedures well, rather than encourage attempts at difficult excisions and repairs. They include sessions on instrumentation, stitchcraft, and cryosurgery. At the annual meetings of the British Association of Dermatologists there are now regular sessions devoted to dermatological surgery organized by the British Dermatological Surgery Group, and including papers on research topics as well as practical procedures.

PROCEDURES – 'HOW TO DO IT'

Conditions

Ideally these should incorporate a full operating suite with trained nursing staff and equipment. It is possible to make do with less, and some excellent work is done in distinctly inferior surroundings, but especially in establishing a new approach I feel it is best to forestall criticism and avoid problems. Most hospitals have one or two free sessions in a suitable theatre and the assistance of trained staff, the facilities for diathermy and suction far outweigh the medicopolitical effort needed to lay claim to these advantages.

Of course all these facilities may be available already within a given dermatology department but this would not be the rule in the UK. Sterile instruments and aseptic procedures are a *sine qua non* for most procedures. Any mistakes in this area can lead to devastating consequences. I scrub and gown for all but the most trivial of tasks.

Anaesthesia

This should be local and not general in the vast majority of cases. Even quite large and lengthy procedures can be performed with adequate local anaesthesia. In general this should be lignocaine with adrenaline. The usual ampoule in the very convenient dental syringe is 2%, and this is fine for small lesions. However, larger volumes are required for other procedures and then 0.5–1% lignocaine should be used.

To ensure good haemostasis and procure a longer effect adrenaline should be used also – if so the maximum safe volume of lignocaine can be increased by a factor of just over *two*. In general the maximum *amount* of plain lignocaine is 7 mg/kg body weight. This means that approximately 20 ml of 2% lignocaine with 1:80 000 adrenaline is the maximum safe dose for a 70 kg adult. A simple chart has been designed, which is a useful guide to the safe amount of lignocaine in different concentrations (Kelly and Henderson, 1983).

The incidence of allergic reactions to lignocaine is very low, and it does not cross-react with other commonly used -caine anaesthetics such as cinchocaine, benzocaine or procaine.

A longer-acting anaesthetic is bupivacaine (Marcain) which is particularly useful in anaesthetizing donor sites for split skin grafts. The maximum safe dose for a 70 kg adult is 150 mg, with or without adrenaline, i.e. 30 ml of a 0.5% solution.

Sedation

The best and safest sedative is a quiet confident manner, an unhurried demeanour, and small talk. The conversation should include the patient where possible. Intravenous or sublingual diazepam or other drugs are quite unnecessary if the right psychological atmosphere is created. Sudden or unexpected movements and loud noises are to be avoided. With children even the sweetest words may fail, and recourse must be had to premedication or even general anaesthesia, but for normal, or even nervous, elderly adults a simpler approach is usually possible and preferred.

Skin preparation

No perfect procedure is available, but even simple washing with soap and water will reduce the bacterial surface count considerably, and preparations such as 0.05% chlorhexidine will reduce it even more. This chemical antiseptic wash is probably one of the best available, and is useful either in spirit or aqueous solution. If diathermy is to be used the aqueous solution should always be used, and the same for cleaning the skin around the eyes to avoid stinging.

Towelling

Towelling the patient is an art in itself and will simply reflect the good sense and requirements of the individual operator. We would, however, especially commend the square and triangle technique for the face, as one very suitable for isolating the bacteria laden hair and scalp (Figure 1.1).

Practice

All procedures can and should be practised on cadavers, volunteers or pigs' trotters. The latter are in use world-wide in dermatological surgery workshops, and time has amply proved their worth in help-

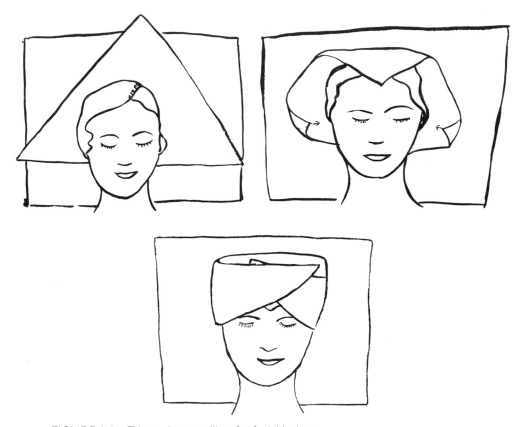

FIGURE 1.1   Triangular towelling for facial lesions

ing the tyro to understand flaps and incisions, and to practise suture techniques.

Emergencies

In over 20 years' busy dermatological and skin surgery practice I have yet to encounter a serious allergic reaction or anaphylaxis to lignocaine. Neither have I yet had to call in colleagues from other specialities to extricate me from embarrassments such as uncontrolled bleeding or severed vital nerves. I believe this is due not entirely to good fortune, but also to careful selection of cases; in particular avoiding problems beyond my capacity; to careful study of the anatomy of the part to be operated on the following day; and to my insistence on having good working conditions and skilled nursing assistance.

Nevertheless it would be reckless to imply that emergencies need not be considered by the skin surgeon. Of these anaphylaxis is probably the most dramatic and life-threatening. Always have available, therefore, adrenaline 1:1000, an antihistamine such as chlorpheniramine for i.v. use, and hydrocortisone 100 mg for i.v. use.

These drugs should be given in that order in cases of anaphylaxis; the adrenaline up to 1 ml slowly subcutaneously, intramuscularly or even i.v. in the most dire cases. The hydrocortisone takes longest to act (up to 30 min) and is most useful in protecting against the sequelae of anaphylaxis.

Oxygen should be administered and an adequate airway maintained. External cardiac massage may be necessary, and cardiac electrostimulation in cases of ventricular fibrillation or standstill.

With these procedures effectiveness derives from forethought and training.

Toxic effects of local anaesthetics can usually be controlled with oxygen, i.v. diazepam or i.v. barbiturates such as sodium thiopentone.

Haemorrhage is generally controllable by the usual measures of clipping, sutures and diathermy. Scalp bleeding may be troublesome but fortunately direct pressure on the calvarium is effective until precise localization and ligation can be achieved. Large vessels in the axillae are only encountered in thin patients, e.g. during Shelley's operation, and should be treated with great respect – especially the veins, which are more vulnerable than the thick-walled arteries. The two vital precepts are, as always:

1. Never cut where you can't see.
2. Never cut what you can't identify.

Following these precepts should also protect important nerves, such as:

1. the facial nerve (especially the mandibular branch) as it emerges from the anterior surface of the parotid gland;

2. the spinal accessory nerve which runs across the posterior triangle of the neck – this innervates the trapezius and damage may lead to permanent dropped shoulder;
3. the common peroneal nerve in the lateral popliteal space as it gives rise to the superficial peroneal nerve.

If these nerves are accidentally severed they should be repaired if necessary by a plastic or neurosurgeon.

Procedures

Simple excision and biopsy techniques

These are among the commonest procedures practised by dermatologists, and yet they are sometimes performed so badly that I feel a detailed guide is justified. Indeed, it was seeing the end-results of such small operations performed by a series of house officers and registrars that initially convinced the author of the need for more formal tuition of dermatological surgery to junior dermatologists in training.

The first task is to choose the area to be biopsied (if not the total excision of a lesion). This should be an obviously active and preferably fairly new part of the rash or lesion. In special cases clinically uninvolved skin is required – e.g. as in the immunofluorescent studies of bullous diseases like dermatitis herpetiformis or pemphigoid. Next, the direction of the long axis of the biopsy should be chosen if this is of the conventional fusiform (sometimes mis-called elliptical) shape.

The older ideas of Langer's lines are now virtually abandoned; the key to success is to choose a long axis parallel to crease marks – or even in the crease marks – if available. That way least tension is produced upon the suture line and the least unattractive scar will form. Crease marks are best identified by pinching and rolling and manipulating the skin under the fingers. If there is still doubt it is perfectly in order to perform a circular excision (most tumours and lesions in dermatology are roughly circular), and observe which way the circle re-forms into an oval – then suture the long edges of the oval together, and repair the dog-ears which will usually be left at either end of the wound (see repair of dog-ears) (Figure 1.2).

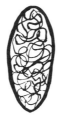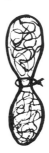

FIGURE 1.2   Circular excision of lesion

Obviously in old patients (especially in light damaged skin) it is easy to choose crease marks, and the cosmetic results of surgery are usually excellent, especially on the face. This is not true, unfortunately, of young patients, who have few creases; thick, active collagen and fibroblasts; and produce more prominent scarring.

The exact lines of the proposed cuts are carefully drawn with a pen and Bonney's Blue, or a felt-tip skin marker. Local anaesthetic is then injected slowly and carefully in sufficient quantities to fully anaesthetize the area to be excised and to allow for any expected undercutting laterally. The usual ratio of length to width is 2.5–3.0 to 1.0, otherwise dog-ears will result. These can, however, be repaired fairly easily (see later).

The incision should be made clearly and firmly, beginning at one end with the blade held vertically, then sloping it so as to use the belly of the blade as progress is made along the length of the wound, reverting to the vertical as the extreme end is reached. A similar wound is made the other side, avoiding cross-hatching of the two lines. The blade can also be sloped a little away from the lesion; this will ensure greater bulk of tissue at the wound edges and tend to produce the slight eversion of the suture line which leads to quickest and most cosmetic healing. The depth of tissue cut depends on the size of lesion to be removed, its own depth and the thickness of the local skin.

As far as possible an even depth should be aimed at to result in a regular even suture line and contour.

Over important structures such as the facial nerve and temporal blood vessels, 5–10 ml normal saline should be injected to raise the skin and lesion away from these structures. This also helps haemostasis and will convert a loose floppy tissue such as lips or ear-lobes into firm tense material which can be more readily manipulated and cut. It is a particularly useful technique in performing a *vermilionectomy* (lip shave).

Undermining or undercutting is a useful manoeuvre where there is some difficulty in bringing the edges of a wound together without tension (Figure 1.3). Tension is to be avoided as much as possible,

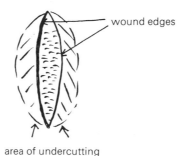

FIGURE 1.3   Undercutting around fusiform excision

as it contributes to poor wound healing, suture marks and possible wound dehiscence when the skin sutures are removed. Gentle undermining with curved, blunt-ended scissors or the scalpel should be done especially along the middle of the wound where tension is likely to be greatest. Opening the scissor blades is almost as useful as cutting with them, and is certainly a good deal safer. Two important points: (1) never cut where you cannot see; (2) never cut any structure you have not identified. No apologies for repetition! It is often helpful and certainly less traumatic to skin edges to use skin hooks rather than toothed forceps which may crush tissue, during the stages of undercutting and suturing. Particularly if undermining has been judged necessary, and often anyway, it is sound practice to insert absorbable subcuticular/subcutaneous sutures. This has two functions: (1) to eliminate any dead space which could accumulate blood and serum and encourage infection; (2) to appose the skin edges so as to permit skin sutures to be placed without tension, or not at all – their function being served by application of adhesive tapes. Any ugly 'railway-track' suture marks are thereby avoided.

If subcuticular sutures are correctly used the function of the skin sutures is purely cosmetic, and they should not be under any significant tension at all. In general they should be inverted, i.e. the knot is buried deep in the tissue by inserting the suture deep, and ending deep (Figure 1.4a,b). In this way the sometimes dark-coloured suture will be invisible at the surface, and 'spitting' (extrusion) of suture material over the weeks ahead is less likely. Needless patient anxiety is thus avoided.

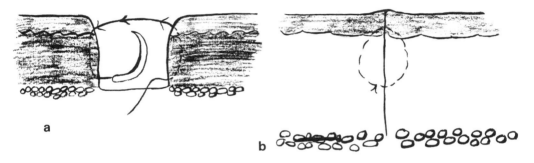

FIGURE 1.4   Buried subcuticular suture

The usual material for subcuticular interrupted sutures is *Dexon* (polyglycolic acid) or *Vicryl* (polyglactin-910). Dexon retains 50% of its strength for about 10 days and disssolves completely in 90–120 days. It causes little tissue reaction and is much stronger than catgut, which is being used less and less. Vicryl is stronger than Dexon and ties more easily. Gauges from 2/O to 5/O are suitable for most dermatological surgery. Subcuticular sutures must be inserted solidly into dermal collagen, not just subdermal fat, which has no anchoring properties. Sutures must be inserted through fat, however, to eliminate dead spaces. The hallmark of the competent dermatological surgeon is the insertion of a really neat continuous subcuticular suture line (Figures 1.5 and 1.6). This is usually of prolene (polypropylene) and should obviate the need for skin sutures altogether,

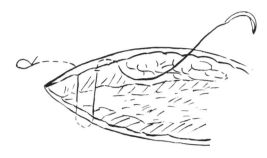

FIGURE 1.5   Continuous subcuticular suture

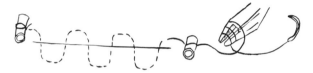

FIGURE 1.6   Continuous subcuticular suture

giving the best cosmetic result of any available technique. It should not be used where there is significant tension between the wound edges.

The *skin sutures* should be of nylon, prolene or some such strong monofilament. Braided threads should be avoided, for although easier to tie they encourage infection, probably by capillary action. The tendency of knots to slip with the monofilament sutures can be avoided by throwing an extra loop into the knot, and by painting the suture line with Whitehead's varnish or collodion. Silk is the most satisfactory of all threads to tie, but is weak, causes inflammation, and apart from special sites such as eyelids, lips or penis, is rapidly being replaced by the modern synthetic threads.

Skin sutures should be placed neatly and evenly spaced, and ideally be 'flask-shaped' in profile (Figure 1.7a,b). This will produce a slight bunch-up of tissue and eversion of the suture line, which is ideal for quick healing and good cosmesis. Inversion of the suture line is accompanied by slow healing and permanent depression with shadowing. The first two or three throws of the thread should be in one direction, the next one or two should be in the opposite direction, and the next one or two in the original direction once

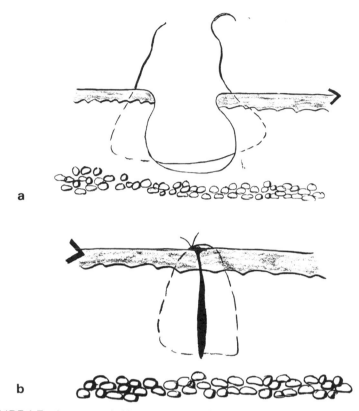

FIGURE 1.7   Interrupted skin suture; note 'flask-shape' in profile

more. 'Square knots' are thus tied, not 'grannies' which tend to slip. Crossing the wrists at the first and third throws automatically pulls the threads in the correct direction.

In general the bites of tissue should be equal either side of the wound, unless one wishes deliberately to elevate one side. The first throw should be lightly tied, the next more tightly, and the third tightest – but not so tight as to totally strangulate all the enclosed tissue. 'If it's white it's too tight' is a little maxim preached at all dermatological surgery workshops throughout the world.

The needles should, of course, be atraumatic – i.e., swaged on to the suture and reverse-cutting wherever possible. This is to avoid cutting the tissue next to the wound. The gauge for skin work is from 2/O for limbs and trunk to 7/O for eyelids and lips.

13

The most generally useful forceps are *Adson's*, which are not too springy, are solid-feeling, and toothed or non-toothed. The former are more generally useful, but the latter are less traumatizing to tissue and useful in helping to evert edges of wound at the end of an operation. It is sometimes difficult to achieve eversion of skin edges with simple interrupted sutures, so that mattress sutures either vertical or horizontal are useful (Figure 1.8a,b). They can be alternated

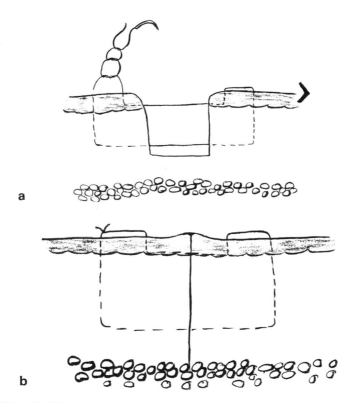

FIGURE 1.8   Vertical mattress suture

with simple interrupted or just three or four placed at appropriate intervals along the suture line. They also reduce the tension on the skin edges, and if this is significant some sort of buttress may be required against the skin surface, e.g. rubber tubing, paraffin gauze or even pieces from the cardboard packet of the suture itself.

All bleeding points must be identified and either diathermied or tied before closure. Careful inspection underneath flaps is essential in regard to this. Small vessels often stop bleeding spontaneously or after squeezing and twisting with artery forceps. Do not be too free with diathermy, especially near nerves, as damaging current may run for a certain length along these structures causing considerable damage even at a distance. Large amounts of charred tissue also make for slow healing and increased risk of infection. Bipolar coagulaters are much kinder to tissues, though they require more precision in their application. In general vessels greater than 1 mm in diameter should be tied not diathermied.

Dressings

I use iodoform compound paint (Whitehead's varnish) on most wounds, but not near the eye because of irritation. This has two functions: one, it is a good antiseptic; and the other, it secures knots. Even well-tied square knots sometimes slip with modern monofilament sutures. Whitehead's varnish also helps adhesive tapes to remain securely on the skin, either at the end of the operation or subsequently at the time of suture removal. The wound can be left open and washed gently after 48 hours, covered with a genuinely non-adherent dressing, e.g. Johnson and Johnson N.A. dressing. There is still controversy over the optimal management of wounds, but the consensus is that occlusion accelerates healing but also encourages infection. Really clean wounds are best occluded, therefore, and suspect ones left open.

Removal of sutures

This is almost as important as their insertion. The *timing* of removal depends upon site, age and state of patient, size of wound, amount of tension and type of sutures. Of these factors *site* is the most critical. With face wounds 4–5 days is sufficient, and 3–4 days in the case of eyelids. With scalp and upper limb wounds 7–8 days; with trunk and lower limb wounds, up to 2 weeks. If subcuticular sutures are taking the strain, the surface sutures can be removed earlier. Removal is best done after cleaning with 0.5% chlorhexidine using fine, sharp-pointed scissors (iris scissors) and Adson's or Whitfield's forceps. So-called suture removal blades and plastic forceps are quite useless. The knot or suture end should be pulled *towards the line of the wound* and then the loop cut flush with the skin. If the knot is pulled away from the edge this puts strain on the healing tissue and the wound might dehisce immediately or later. If there is any doubt about the security of the wound remove alternate sutures and replace them with adhesive tapes. The remaining sutures can be removed then or several days later. Removal of the adhesive strips is best done by lifting both ends *simultaneously* and pulling gently towards the wound edge.

The actual healing and remodelling process continues in the dermis for several months and patients should be encouraged to treat this area gently when washing and drying the skin.

Large excisions, e.g. for malignant tumours, may produce problems in closure. The point to establish here is that in the last resort it is simply not necessary to close most wounds at the time of operation to get perfectly good healing and acceptable cosmetic results. Nature takes care of such open wounds very well, providing they are cleansed thoroughly once daily, with a mild antiseptic such as 0.5% chlorhexidine (or even soap and water). They take longer to heal, and in general most patients will require daily dressing but they can quite readily be done at home by the patient if necessary. Surprisingly many originally circular or oval wounds heal to produce a fine linear scar, presumably because of the interplay of muscular and other forces on the dermis. This can be assisted by inserting guiding sutures once every 7-10 days so as to ensure the eventual linear scar is in the optimal direction (Figure 1.9). Any unpleasant cosmetic residue can be excised or refashioned at a later date. Dermabrasion is useful in smoothing down ugly or irregular scars in this respect. Most plastic surgeons have a professional pride in filling in holes, but endorsement of allowing healing by secondary intention comes from very distinguished schools and is soundly based in physiology and anatomy. Some areas should be avoided, however – e.g. too close to the edge of the eyelids, above an eyebrow, close to the lip, as ectropion or other unacceptable deformity may ensue. Usually

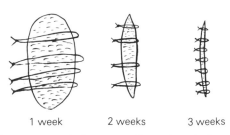

FIGURE 1.9 Guiding suture technique over 3-week period

even these results can be adequately corrected at a later stage. The advantages of open healing are:

1. the operation is quicker, easier for the patient, and can be performed with relative ease by someone of modest surgical skills;
2. further surgery is simple if the histologist reports incomplete removal of a malignant tumour, whereas grafts and flaps would have to be undone and refashioned;
3. it is the basis of the Mohs' technique, now accepted as the most certain way of fully excising malignant tissue of the skin;
4. infection and haemorrhage rarely present problems.

When removing a tumour, either using Mohs' technique or by simple excision, it is often useful to place a marking suture at a given point (usually 12 o'clock) to help the pathologist orientate the specimen (this is, of course, unnecessary in the subsequent steps of the Mohs' technique as the edges of the specimens are painted).

Flaps and grafts

Closure can also be accomplished by using (a) flaps, (b) free grafts.

Flap repairs from surrounding normal skin, if properly designed and executed, give excellent cosmetic results because they fill the defect with skin of similar colour and texture. There is a large number of different flap repairs and only the simpler ones will be recommended here. The simplest of all is the bilateral bipedal flap – which translated is simply the execution of generous undermining of the edges of a simple fusiform (so-called elliptical) excision.

Next is the V–Y flap, which is often useful on lower leg wounds, which often spring open to alarming proportions after the excision of quite a modest sample of skin! It is also useful above an eyebrow (to prevent elevation of the eyebrow), and on the back of the hands. This technique relaxes the main wound, and can be single, bilateral and multiple. The open end of the V should be placed about $\frac{1}{2}$–1 cm away from the main wound, the V converted to a Y as the main wound is sutured, and the junction of the dermis and stem of the Y closed using a three-point suture (Figure 1.10). This must not be too tight or necrosis of the tip of skin between the limbs of the Y will occur. This is a pity because one of the very reasons for performing a flap repair is to avoid tension and consequent necrosis.

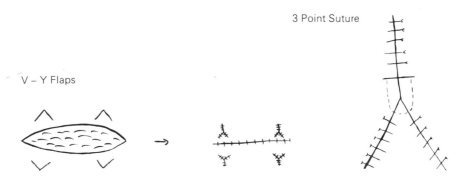

FIGURE 1.10   V–Y flaps following fusiform excision of lesion, showing three-point suture technique

Simple advancement flaps

This is a useful technique in many situations, especially on the trunk and limbs, and on the nose. Here the Burow's triangle is helpful to ensure adequate movement of the flap and to avoid bunching up of tissue at the base of the pedicle (Figure 1.11). The ratio of breadth to length should be 1:1 or 1:1.5 on the trunk and lower limb, 1:2 on the upper limb, but may be 1:2.5 or even 1:3 on the well-vascularized face. These are proportions of so-called *random pattern flaps*, but flaps containing a well-defined axis of blood vessels (axial pattern flap) may be much longer in relation to their width. Undercutting, mobilization, and the creation of Burow's triangles are often necessary in flap formation. Meticulous haemostasis and avoidance of

Single advancement flap

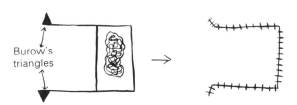

FIGURE 1.11   Single advancement flap with Burow's triangle

infection and tension are also absolute requirements for flaps to survive. Blanching indicates tension and may indicate a non-viable flap. Free split-skin grafts can be used to cover defects produced by the formation of the flap of full-thickness skin. Firm but not too tight pressure bandaging is a useful aid in preventing haematoma and seroma formation post-operatively.

Double advancement flaps

Double advancement flaps (H-plasties) are particularly useful on the forehead and eyebrows, so as to avoid elevation of eyebrows and other deformities in removing tumours. As usual, incisions are placed in crease marks wherever possible (Figure 1.12).

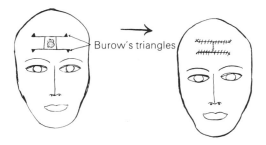

FIGURE 1.12   Double advancement flap or H-plasty

19

Transposition flaps

These are very useful in the nasolabial region, and for closing defects on the side of the nose. The skin of the cheek is an excellent match, and the blood supply so good that length/base ratios of 3:1 are usually successful. Similar flaps can be used to cover defects of the lateral lower eyelid using skin from the upper eyelid. Again it must be emphasized that *total excision* of a malignancy must be ensured before such closures are undertaken.

O–Z plasties

These are of wide application. They really consist of two rotation flaps (Figure 1.13); Burow's triangles are usually necessary to accomplish closure without tension. The central limb of the Z must be placed so as to fall into, or parallel with, a natural crease or wrinkle.

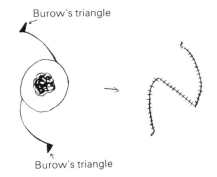

Burow's triangle

Burow's triangle

FIGURE 1.13   O–Z plasty technique

This closure is a natural sequence following circular excisions of tumours, a useful technique when it is not clear where the natural lines of tension are. After circular excision the defect usually assumes an oval form, with the long axis along the line of tension and where a natural crease might be expected to develop in the course of aging.

The rotation flap

This is simple, and usually successful because of its broad pedicle (Figure 1.14). The defect can be either triangulated or circular. If closure is difficult bilateral rotation flaps can be constricted, so that an A to T flap results (Figure 1.15).

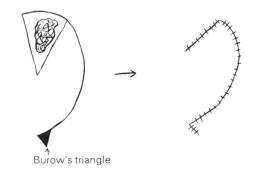

Burow's triangle

FIGURE 1.14   Rotation flap following triangular excision of lesion

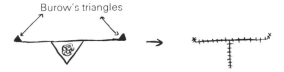

Burow's triangles

FIGURE 1.15   A–T flap technique (A is inverted in this illustration)

M-plasty

M-plasty is used where it is desirable to shorten a wound (Figure 1.16). The M can be bilateral or at one end of an excision; e.g. to avoid a structure such as ala nasi, or vermilion border of lip.

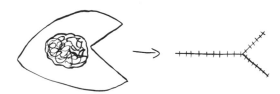

FIGURE 1.16   M-plasty

Z-plasty

This procedure is of value in reducing tension along a wound or established scar. It relieves this and switches any remaining tension along a different direction (Figure 1.17).

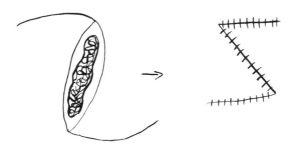

FIGURE 1.17   Z-plasty technique; note alteration of main axis

The angle between the lines of the Z are classically at 60° to the central bar but smaller angles (down to 30°) are frequently used, and this produces *less* lengthening of original wound or scar. Multiple Z-plasties can be constructed along a wound or after excising a contracted scar both to release tension and to break up the linear wound into smaller, less visible sections.

Some general notes on flaps

The purposes of flaps are (1) to cover defects with similar-looking local skin, and (2) to reduce tension. The most frequent question asked at Workshops about flaps is – 'when should I use such-and-such a flap?'. The answer is:

1. Wherever you have produced a defect which you cannot close primarily without significant tension, and which you therefore wish to close with well-matched skin taken from the same locality which can spare it. In general the cosmetic results of flaps are superior to free grafts and healing by secondary intention.
2. The simpler and more broad-based the flap, the likelier it is to succeed. Narrow-based flaps on the trunk or limbs will die at the

distal end through ischaemia unless they are based on a known substantial vascular component.

Therefore on the trunk and limbs, random flaps (i.e. not based on known vascular components) should not have greater than 1:1 or 1:1.5 breadth to length ratio. Often this means that advancement and rotation flaps are the commonly used flaps for these sites. On the face and neck the blood supply is much better, and random flaps with ratios of 1:3 or even 1:4 breadth to length are commonly achieved. Here the transposition flaps are extremely useful – for nose, eyelids and in front of the ear.

Points of technique

Considerable undercutting is nearly always required to mobilize flaps. The depth at which this is carried out depends on the site; on the face and neck it should be very superficial – about 3 mm below the skin surface, though this may be a little thicker on the forehead. The aim is to provide a piece of tissue which one can work with, but to avoid cutting underlying structures such as vessels and nerves. On the scalp the least vascular place is below the galea and superficial to the periosteum. On the proximal limb and trunk the flaps will consist of skin plus superficial fascia.

Subcuticular suturing is usually desirable and it is helpful to place one or two anchoring sutures at key points (which can be removed later) to guide repair.

Avoidance of *tension*, haemorrhage, and infection are the keys to successful repair.

Free grafts

These may be (1) split skin grafts (SSG or Thiersch grafts); (2) full-thickness grafts (FTG or Wolfe grafts).

Split skin grafting (SSG)

This procedure is easy to perform with practice. Nearly always the grafts take well, even on relatively poorly vascularized or even infected sites such as leg ulcers. SSGs tend to shrink, especially if very thin, and never develop the bulk of FTGs so that they are unsuitable for areas such as soles and palms. The donor site is always visible and may cover a considerable area.

Many grafting knives are available; the small Silver dermatome is useful for small procedures and is found in many Accident Departments. I favour the Braithwaite modification of the Humby knife; with experience one can gauge the depth of skin taken quite accurately, and for a research project some years ago I was able to take specimens consisting of 90–95% epidermis from the skin over the upper back using this instrument.

The technique is best learned from watching an experienced surgeon at work. Practice on oranges, pigs' trotters and cadavers can also be helpful. The main faults are; (a) uneven sweep so that skin of varying thickness is obtained, and an ugly scar; and (b) specimens which are too thick – in effect almost FTG. This is unfortunate as it means the donor skin may not flourish, and because the donor site will not heal. If this is recognized at the time of operation some small pieces of graft should be spared if possible, and replaced onto the central donor site. The fault is recognized not only by observing the thickness of the specimen but also by noting the comparative paucity of the normally numerous dermal papillary blood vessels cut in a well-performed procedure. If necessary a separate small *thinner* graft should be taken from another site (e.g. deltoid) to cover the full-thickness deficiency. If the operator pauses after 1–2 cm has been cut he will see if his setting is correct for that particular patient's skin. It is of course vital not to place the graft on upside-down – not easy to do with large single grafts, but quite possible with postage stamp-size grafts such as often advocated for leg ulcers. Meshing the graft with a special machine increases the area feasible to cover, and also decreases infection and increases 'take' rate. This probably works well as there is free drainage between the pieces of grafted skin, as with the postage stamp-size grafts.

The usual donor site is upper inner thigh, but the deltoid region, the upper inner arm, the back, or the buttock, can also be suitable sources. The selected area should be fully anaesthetized with lignocaine, or better, 0.25% Marcain with 1:400 000 adrenaline. Up to 150 mg (60 ml) of this long-acting anaesthetic can be safely used for the average 70 kg adult.

In taking the graft the skin must be steadied at one end by an assistant using a wooden grafting board, and a paraffin-lubricated board is held by the operator and moved steadily and firmly in front of the moving knife which is also lightly lubricated on the roller knife edge. A steady horizontal sawing motion should be aimed at, not irregular digs vertically. At the end of the cut the blade should be angled upwards, and this will automatically cut the end of the specimen.

The donor site should be covered after cleansing with 0.5% aqueous chlorhexidine with an adhesive dressing such as OP-site. This membrane is a gas-permeable polyethylene film with an adhesive backing, which allows free movement of oxygen, carbon dioxide and water vapour, while excluding larger molecules and bacteria. It dramatically decreases the pain and discomfort – previously the norm with donor sites   and healing, if anything, is enhanced. Blood and serum which accumulate beneath the film can be drained by incising the film under aseptic conditions every 48 hours.

The graft itself should be fixed in position with interrupted fine sutures e.g. 4/O or 5/O Ethilon. The graft should overlap the edge of the defect (Figure 1.18) and there is no need to trim these edges; they will dry up and shrink to the edge over the ensuing days. Two or three basting sutures are helpful in the centre of the graft to eliminate slippage, and prevent 'tenting' with blood and serum. A tie-over pressure dressing using eyepads or sponges gives the final security. The tie-over sutures of 2/O or 3/O nylon are placed at quadrants of the graft, left long, and tied over the dressing firmly but not so tight as to impede vascularization. The causes of failure of SSG are:

1. bleeding,
2. infection,
3. accumulation of serum under the graft separating it from its bed,
4. slippage of graft on site.

Only meticulous attention paid to avoiding these complications will ensure a high success rate.

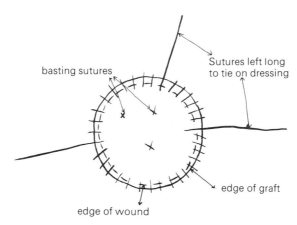

FIGURE 1.18   Split skin graft; note basting sutures and overlapping of wound edges

The recipient site and graft need not be inspected until suture removal on about the 10th day. During this period ideally the part should be elevated and rested. The grafted site may need to be inspected if there is undue pain (most unusual) or pyrexia, indicating the presence of infection. At suture removal it is not uncommon to see some detachment of epidermis, or even small areas of sloughing. Do not decide too early that the graft has failed. Careful cleansing, replacement of dressings, topical antiseptics and systemic and/or topical antibiotics may save even a very unpromising-looking situation.

SSG is the closure of choice for large defects, e.g. after excision of malignant melanoma. They are especially useful with malignancies in general, as recurrences can be detected more readily under an SSG than a thicker FTG, or a flap. The latter have the additional disadvantage of distorting tissue planes so that recurrences may lie undetected, sometimes for considerable periods before their eventual discovery. This is one of the main reasons for insisting on total excision of malignant tissue before flap repairs.

Contraindications to SSG
These are:

1. weight-bearing areas, or areas subject to repeated friction trauma;
2. facial defects – though this is not an absolute bar, and certainly not in regard to malignant melanomas.

Full-thickness grafts (FTG)

These have a better cosmetic appearance than SSG, though not so good as a well-designed flap. The donor site must be closed, either by primary suture or an SSG. Such grafts do not shrink much after excision, nor contract in the long term *in situ*.

Well-chosen donor sites can give excellent colour and texture matches for the recipient area, e.g. retro-auricular skin for eyelids and upper cheek; upper eyelid skin to lower eyelid; nasolabial fold to side of nose; and neck to face. Obviously account must be taken of the amount and direction of hair growth, pigmentation, vascularity and thickness, in deciding what is a suitable donor site.

Once decided upon the donor site should be drawn out precisely to the size and shape of the recipient site to be filled.

A template of X-ray film, cardboard from a suture package, or even gauze pressed on the recipient site is helpful, though precise measurements with a ruler are preferred by some. Allowance for a little immediate shrinkage say 3–5 mm in a 5 cm diameter graft should be made. The graft should be trimmed of fat and then sutured carefully in place *without overlapping*, using 4/O or 5/O prolene or nylon sutures. A tie-over dressing, as with SSG, may be used also. Secure fixation with a firm dressing should then be done, and the part elevated if possible. Sutures are removed at 7–10 days for both donor and recipient sites.

Never take the graft before cutting out the lesion, as the recipient area always expands somewhat once the natural skin tension is relieved by excising the central area.

It is better to overestimate the amount of skin required in repairing lower eyelid defects, as ectropion is otherwise all too readily produced, requiring further and more difficult correction later.

The scalp rarely needs grafting. Even quite large defects can be repaired by primary suture providing adequate undermining in the sub-aponeurotic layer has been performed. This is amply proved by scalp reduction techniques as practised for male pattern alopecia (MPA) where excision and primary suture of strips 10×2.5–3.0 cm are commonplace.

Punch grafts as used in male pattern baldness are a special type of

FTG. They take well and if skilfully executed can produce quite cosmetically acceptable results nowadays.

Careful attention to details of direction of hair growth and marginal line are essential to good work. The pioneering work of Norman Orentreich, a New York dermatologist in the 1960s, ushered in a new era in the management of MPA, and though Juri flaps and scalp reduction surgery have to some extent replaced punch grafting, it still remains a safe and useful technique for many types of MPA, both as the main treatment and to supplement the more major procedures. Up to 600 plugs can be taken at one sitting, though the usual number is 100–150. An electric drill is commonly used nowadays, as the operator's fingers soon become fatigued.

Curettage

Curettage is surely one of the most versatile techniques, as well as the most undervalued or even derided technique, in the dermatologist's armamentarium. In fact properly used, a sharp curette can deal not only with common warts, pyogenic granulomas, keratoacanthomas, and the like, but also basal cell carcinomas in a very adequate fashion. Indeed 5-year cure rates of up to 95% have been published using curettage and diathermy. The emphasis is, of course, on 'properly used' – for much worse results may be produced by inexperienced junior staff. In North America the ring curette is favoured, whereas in the UK the solid spoon type of instrument is generally used. I have little doubt, however, that the hollow ring type is superior in practically all cases. Unless the curette is exceedingly sharp it is useful to circle the area to be curetted with a small No. 11 or No. 15 scalpel blade before inserting the curette. In the case of basal cell carcinomas the curettage is followed by the cautery or electro-desiccation, and then a second curettage is performed to remove the charred tissue and to explore any small soft channels or 'runs' of malignant tissue which can be discovered. A final cauterization or electro-desiccation is then performed to achieve haemostasis. Alternatively this may be achieved by applying trichloracetic acid (60–90%), aluminium chloride 50% in alcohol, 80% phenol or Monsel's solution (ferric subsulphate).

Dermabrasion

This was a technique invented by a dermatologist (Kromayer), used extensively by dermatologists for some years, and then taken over by plastic surgeons, at least in the UK. It is a valuable technique for improving some scars, either elevated or depressed, mild rhinophymas, and certain tattoos; it can also help the multiple fine wrinkles of aged skin. Most plastic surgeons use general anaesthetic, but this really compels the operator to be fairly radical in his approach. I prefer to do multistage dermabrasion, under local anaesthetic, and this way can gauge the effect and amend technique according to the response of the patient. I routinely use the Stryker instrument, and have done so for many years.

Many dermatologists use local freezing sprays containing Freon and other gases under pressure; this freezes the skin, ensures a bloodless field, and gives the patient some moderate analgesia. I suspect the inflammatory reaction following fairly thorough freezing is also therapeutically helpful in many cases. Certainly the woody-hard frozen skin is easy to work with, and the absence of blood is an advantage except in so far as it is more difficult to judge the depth of the wound in these conditions.

Dermabrasion is not a technique for the tyro or the unwary. Considerable damage may be done within seconds by the rapidly revolving heads of the instrument. Particularly around the eyelids and lips, where there is unsupported tissue, the operator must be especially careful, otherwise very serious damage may be done to these structures.

It is wise to have a sensible assistant holding the skin firmly and isolating the patch being dermabraded from the surrounding tissues. Do not use gauze for this purpose, as there is a risk of it being caught up in the revolving head, whipping around at several thousand revolutions per minute and doing a good deal of damage to nearby structures.

A fine aerosol of blood and skin is evoked during the procedure, some of which may well be inhaled by those working close to the patient. Whether the operator and his assistants wear protective gowns, masks and helmets or not, and even when using a guard for the head, it is mandatory these days to know the hepatitis B and

HTLV-III/LAV status of the patient, and to refuse dermabrasion to positive reactors.

Many scars are *not* suitable for dermabrasion; so-called 'ice-pick' scars in acne – small, deep pits – do not respond well; indeed any really deep, sharp-edged scar does poorly with this technique, and other methods give superior results – e.g. simple excision, and fine suturing or elevation of a round deep scar using a small punch (Figure 1.19).

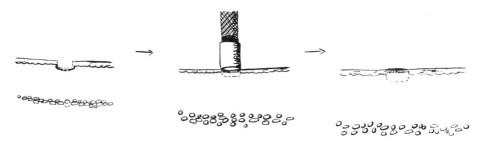

FIGURE 1.19   Removal of 'ice-pick' scar using punch trephine

Special techniques

Horizontal excision of naevi

This is a simple technique giving excellent cosmetic results. Obviously the naevi must be assuredly benign, and this is where an experienced and competent dermatologist has the edge over most other surgeons and physicians, to say nothing of beauticians who also treat moles. The naevus should not be deeply pigmented, since this type of excision may not remove all melanocytes and small seedlings producing dark pigmented spots in the scar produce considerable alarm. Hairy naevi are unsuitable unless the operator is prepared to go back later and remove the hair roots and papillae by electrolysis or diathermy. The naevus is anaesthetized and then simply shaved off horizontally, in the plane of the surrounding skin. The bleeding base is then *lightly* cauterized by diathermy or a chemical styptic such as trichloracetic acid or aluminium chloride. Monsel's solution is also used, and only very rarely produces pigmentation from iron tattooing. The wound is best left open to the air, or painted with Whitehead's varnish and washed gently with an antiseptic twice daily for 1 week.

If the diagnosis is correct the risk of malignancy supervening is to all intents and purposes nil. Throughout the world this technique has been used for many thousand of benign moles over many years, and no malignant change as a result of this technique has ever been reported.

Vermilionectomy

This is well within a dermatological surgeon's capability, and a valuable technique in dealing with actinic keratoses of the lip and actinic cheilitis. It can be combined with simple V-excision of established malignancies of the lip.

The lip is anaesthetized by infiltration, and then 5–10 ml normal saline injected into the lip. This reduces bleeding and produces a firm material much easier to work with than the unexpanded tissue. Sutures (2/O) can be inserted at either end of the lip for the convenience of the assistant, and cut out at the end of the operation. The whole unhealthy area is then excised leaving a raw area 0.5–1.0 cm wide. Haemostasis is secured, and the mucous membrane pattern of the defect brought forward and sutured to the skin. This may (but may not) require some undercutting. If neatly done the patient is left with a normal-looking lip consisting of mucous membrane which soon becomes keratinized, and since it has had little exposure to actinic radiation should last him for 20–30 years.

Repair of dog-ears

This is easily done with sharp-pointed scissors, producing either a longer wound or a shorter one if bipolar M-plasties are performed.

Electrosurgery

In the UK (and in many US practices) this is commonly accomplished using a small diathermy machine, the Hyfrecator. A high-voltage, high-frequency, damped current is applied usually with a monoelectrode to the lesion. A great variety of benign and malignant tumours can be destroyed with this technique. Benign skin papillomas of the neck and axillae (skin tags) respond well, and do not need to be anaesthetized. Spider naevi, small angiomas, and certain telangiectatic lesions of the face and legs also respond well.

The procedure is used extensively in the USA to achieve haemostasis during Mohs' surgery. Small cysts and persistent acne papules also respond well. Trichoepitheliomas of the face and eyelids can easily be removed and the small papules of adenoma sebaceum can be destroyed in this way. Small warts and verrucas will often require anaesthesia and surgical needles are available to perform epilation. This is a very versatile and safe instrument and most dermatologists possess one, though they do not always exploit its full potential.

The hot cautery has more limited application and will produce unpleasant scars if not carefully used. It too can be used for haemostasis, e.g. after curettage of warts and tumours.

Collagen and silicone implants

The current fashion is to use bovine collagen modified chemically to decrease immunogenicity and increase stability. 'Zyderm' is the most popular brand at present, though a cheaper Japanese version is on the market in some countries, and no doubt will be on sale in the UK eventually. Zyderm is extremely expensive (almost £70 for 1 ml), but is undoubtedly an effective agent in reducing certain wrinkles, and elevating some depressed scars. It is of notable help in the very common glabellar frown marks, and the vertical and usually multiple wrinkles of upper and lower lips. A test dose of 0.1 ml is injected intradermally first, and observed over 4 weeks.

A small percentage of patients show an immediate or delayed reaction to this, and cannot be treated. A small number also develop allergic reactions later, and a few have developed generalized immune responses with fever, polyarthropathy and the like. Patients with evidence of collagen vascular disease should obviously not be treated with this material. It is important to overcorrect, as a good deal of the bulk of injected material disappears within a few days. The double-strength Zyderm makes this less necessary, but of course is yet more expensive. Eventually all of the injected foreign collagen is metabolized, but some of the patient's own collagen is laid down, no doubt as a response to the foreign material. This means that although booster injections may be necessary every 6–12 months, they are not usually so large, and not inevitable. The more superficial the injection, the better. A peau d'orange effect is to be aimed at following injection. An unfortunate tendency is for the collagen solution, which is injected under some considerable pressure, to seep out of the sebaceous follicular openings, or along needle tracks. This means that some wastage of very expensive material occurs.

Apart from this irritation, and an allergic reaction developing in one patient, I have so far encountered no snags in using this material over the last 3 years, and in my view it certainly has a place in cosmetic dermatological surgery. If it were cheaper I would use it a lot more. I have no personal experience of silicone injection, but my reading of the literature, and discussion with colleagues who have, indicates that the present grades of silicone fluids are relatively safe, very unlikely to form granulomas, and are also valuable adjuncts in treating certain types of atrophy and depressed scars (Sorrel Resnik, personal communication, 1985).

Face peels

These are performed either with phenol or trichloracetic acid – operators who use phenol sometimes encounter the toxic effect of absorbed phenol; there may be cardiac arrhythmias and the possibility of renal damage. In view of these findings my own practice is to strictly avoid this technique, which in my view cannot be justified for purely cosmetic benefits. Trichloracetic acid seems to have no systemic adverse effects, and certainly in my hands is a useful preparation for a number of cosmetic problems. Most dermatologists will be familiar with its excellent effect on xanthelasma, offering a very superior alternative to excision and suturing, or curettage. The surrounding skin should be protected with petroleum jelly, a steady hand is needed, and precise applications of the fluid using cotton-wool buds. Reflex tearing nearly always occurs, and the operator must be prepared for this with dry cotton-wool swabs. The area should be neutralized with plain tap water – but thoroughly – after about 10–20 seconds; then the treatment is complete. It is wise to do trial areas using as low a concentration as 20% to begin with, as every patient reacts in an individual fashion. Over-treatment may produce unpleasant scars and even ectropion. Any contamination of the eye (this should not be allowed to happen) must be counteracted by immediate irrigation with normal saline.

Trichloracetic acid, in varying dilutions, can also be used to reduce the fine wrinkling of aged skin, to reduce some post-acne scars, and to reduce the erythema of rhinophymas. The patient must be warned that the skin will become inflamed, and that it should be bathed in tepid water every 2–3 hours for 24–48 hours if this is pronounced. Topical and even systemic corticosteroids may on occasions be necessary. As with xanthelasma, test concentrations should be employed first – 10–20% – and the response observed after 2–3 weeks.

TRAINING AND RESEARCH

Training in the UK is by apprenticeship and example. Formal training schemes in dermatological surgery are not yet available. Any aspiring dermatological surgeon is advised to obtain a year's training fellowship in a recognized centre in the USA. Excellent schemes are in progress there, and some helpful and fruitful contacts already exist between centres in this country such as St John's Hospital, London; Newcastle; and the American schools.

Within the next few years it is to be expected that fellowships, lectureships and eventually senior lectureships will be established, and less reliance will have to be imposed on our ever-generous American friends.

The British Dermatological Surgery Group, founded in 1982, is committed to improving training in this subject. It runs annual courses in practical techniques; and workshops, where stitchcraft, excisions, flaps, and cryosurgery are taught. It also publishes a quarterly newsletter.

Each year at the meeting of the British Association of Dermatologists, to which the BDSG is affiliated, there is an academic session on the subject.

In the wider world the BDSG is affiliated to the International Society for Dermatologic Surgery and currently two members of the BDSG committee serve as council members of the international body (one as a board director). In September 1986 the BDSG act as host to the International Society annual meeting, to be held in the UK for the first time, in London. Thus it can be seen that the subject and its devotees have come far in a relatively few years, from virtually nothing to a small thriving national group.

Mohs' surgery is now practised in Newcastle, Truro, and Gloucester. Other centres will undoubtedly see the need for such work and we envisage one such centre in each region eventually. This has implications for money and manpower, which will have to be taken into account in the development generally of dermatology in the UK. This might seem a bad time to advocate expansion in the NHS, but it would also be irresponsible to ignore the great changes going on in the world outside, many of which can be adapted in this country to the advantage of our patients.

The academic content of most dermatological surgery courses is fairly basic, and there is a great opportunity here for British dermatological surgeons to inject a real contribution of their own. Critical appraisals are needed of many different techniques, including the Mohs' technique, and the general scientific approach of British dermatology could be of great benefit in sorting out some of these problems.

THE FUTURE

I think it would be very difficult to stop the expansion and advance of dermatological surgery now. There has been considerable resistance by plastic surgeons in the USA, and to a lesser degree in the UK, but eventually a *modus vivendi* will be accomplished. Of course there will be overlapping of interests and territories, but the rigid demarcation disputes which impede progress in industry are unlikely to do so in medicine. In fact it is at interfaces between subjects that often most progress is achieved – witness the impact of interventional radiology in coronary heart disease, and for that matter, plastic surgery in microvascular techniques.

All subjects, like languages, change – or die, like Latin. There is no room in the modern world for ossification of ideas and disciplines in their original mould. All of the present specialities of medicine arose as splinter groups from the original main disciplines of medicine and surgery. Now the truly general physician or surgeon is practically extinct.

As to whether dermatological surgeons should be trained formally as surgeons before raising a scalpel to the skin, my answer would be that extensive general surgical training could be a waste of valuable time. Dermatological surgery – incorporating scalpel surgery, curettage, cautery, electrosurgery, laser beam therapy, cryosurgery, dermabrasion – is quite specialized enough and different enough from general surgery to merit separate training and consideration.

Every dermatologist in training in the UK can now have the opportunity to develop some practical experience in the techniques described in this chapter. Some of them, we hope, will wish to further their knowledge and expertise and obtain consultant posts eventually where this type of work will form a significant and satisfying part of their life's work.

1. Stegman, S. J., Tromovitch, T. A., and Glogau, R. G. (1982). *Basics of Dermatologic Surgery*. (Chicago/London: Year Book Medical Publishers)
2. McGregor, I. A. (1980) *Fundamental Techniques of Plastic Surgery and their Surgical Applications*, 7th Edn. (Edinburgh: Churchill Livingstone)
3. Stegman, S. J. and Tromovitch, T. A. (1984) *Cosmetic Dermatologic Surgery*. (Chicago/London: Year Book Medical Publishers)
4. Epstein, E. and Epstein, E. Jr. (1984). *Skin Surgery*, 5th Edn. (Springfield, Ill.; Charles C. Thomas)
5. Petres, J. and Hundeiker, M. (1978). *Dermatosurgery*. (Heidelberg, New York; Springer-Verlag)
6. *The Journal of Dermatologic Surgery and Oncology*. Publisher, Perry Robins, MD
7. Kelly, D. A. and Henderson, A. M. (1983). Use of local anaesthetic drugs in hospital practice. *Br. Med. J.*, **286**, 1784

2
LASERS IN DERMATOLOGY

J. A. S. CARRUTH

GENERAL INTRODUCTION

Albert Einstein described the concept of stimulated emission of radiation, which produces coherent laser light, in 1917, but it was not until 1960 that T. H. Maiman, working for the Hughes Research Laboratory, produced the first laser using a synthetic ruby as the lasing medium.

However, since that time laser technology has advanced very rapidly, and a large number of laser systems have been developed with a vast and ever-increasing range of industrial, scientific and military uses. The range of uses is now so great that it has been suggested that when the age in which we live is finally assessed, it will not be known as the atomic or space age, but the age of the laser.

We are only at the beginning of the laser age, but already lasers have, in a number of fields, turned science fiction into science fact.

With the development of each laser its medical applications were researched and several are now in regular clinical use in a wide range of medical and surgical disciplines, and others are being researched and evaluated. The skin provided an excellent 'test model' for these investigations. Much of the early research was with the pulsed ruby laser, which has now largely been replaced for clinical work by the more controllable continuous wave lasers. However, the ruby laser is still used for the treatment of certain pigmented skin lesions and tattoos.

In all medical and surgical fields, lasers should only be used when it can be shown clearly that a particular task can be better performed by laser than by conventional, established techniques, and the words of Dr Leon Goldman, one of the fathers of laser surgery, must never be forgotten: 'If you don't need a laser, don't use one.'

As with any medical device the use of lasers will gradually be established into those indications where a laser is essential, those where it is of great value, indications in which a laser may be of some use and those where lasers are of no value or a positive disadvantage.

Lasers are expensive and, having acquired one, practitioners tend to use them on a wide range of conditions, some of which are unsuitable, to justify the expense. Some of this practice will undoubtedly result in new applications for each laser, but some will result in totally inappropriate usage.

A number of cases of malpractice have already received publicity and, in these, lasers were used either on inappropriate conditions or in an unacceptable manner. With the huge demand for cosmetic surgery, every effort must be made to define accurate guidelines for the safe and appropriate use of lasers in dermatology, as in all other fields of medicine and surgery.

THE LASER

Introduction

A laser (light amplification by stimulated emission of radiation), is a device which produces coherent light: an intense beam of pure, monochromatic light which does not diverge and in which all the light waves are of the same length and travel in phase and in the same direction.

The lasing medium, which may be a solid, liquid or a gas, is contained in the laser tube which has a fully reflective mirror at one end and a partially reflective mirror at the other, which allows access to the laser beam. The name of the laser is taken from the lasing medium, which in most medical lasers is a gas, and the lasing medium also determines the wavelength of the coherent light produced by the laser. The wavelength of the laser light determines its pattern of absorption by body tissues and its effects on them, and this defines the clinical role of the laser. As each laser produces essentially one wavelength, monochromatic light, it has only one main clinical role, and to change role one must change laser.

There is, however, some overlap in roles of the three most commonly used lasers. The carbon dioxide laser is a high-precision, bloodless light scalpel used for incising and excising tissues with the sealing of small blood vessels. The argon laser is used for blood vessel coagulation but can be used to perform slow, thermal tissue destruction at higher power levels, and the neodymium YAG laser is used both for tissue destruction with good haemostasis and for the control of normal and abnormal blood vessels (Table 2.1).

TABLE 2.1   Roles of lasers

	Cutting	Coagulating
Carbon dioxide	+ +	±
Argon	±	+ +
Neodymium YAG	+	+

Lasing

The lasing medium is excited electrically, or in some cases by another high-energy light source, to produce a population inversion of excited/non-excited particles which normally has a great excess in the low-energy state. An excited particle will decay spontaneously to the low-energy ground state with the release of a photon – a quantum of radiation energy or light particle. If this photon strikes another particle of the lasing medium in the high-energy state, it stimulates it to emit an identical photon, A large number of photons are generated by these collisions and are reflected back into the lasing medium from the mirrors with a rapid build-up of light energy in the laser tube – the cascade effect. The coherent light can then be emitted through the partially reflective mirror to the tissues via a number of delivery systems.

Delivery systems

Both the argon and neodymium YAG laser energy can be transmitted via flexible fibre optic delivery systems which can then be attached to an operating microscope, slit lamp, endoscope delivery fibre or handpiece in the case of the argon laser. The neodymium YAG laser is used with the operating microscope, endoscopic delivery fibre and handpiece which may incorporate a quartz or diamond scalpel blade.

The carbon dioxide laser beam cannot, at present, be transmitted via a flexible fibre, although a number of fibres are being investigated. Delivery of the laser energy to microscope, colposcope or handpiece is via an articulated arm which is a hollow tube with mirrors at the articulations. The beam can be focused to a point using a concave mirror providing high energy levels.

Laser energy

The following treatment parameters must be recorded for each laser treatment:

1. power – the power output measured by the laser or a separate power level meter;
2. power density – power per unit area calculated from the output power of the laser and the size of the laser imprint;
3. energy delivered – a measurement of power/unit time/unit area (Joules/cm^2).

Laser-tissue interaction

It is said that laser energy at low levels may be biostimulative but at higher levels the effects become inhibitory and after this the effects on tissues are thermal. The first thermal effect is to cause cell death followed by coagulation of tissues and ultimately vaporization. In an attempt to make laser therapy more selective the use of photosensitizers is being researched and, at present, haematoporphyrin derivative is used to photosensitize malignant tissues to red laser light produced by a dye or gold vapour laser in the treatment of many forms of localized malignant disease by photoradiation therapy.

LASERS USED CLINICALLY

Argon

The argon laser (Figure 2.1) produces blue/green coherent light at a number of wavelengths but 80% of the energy is at wavelengths of

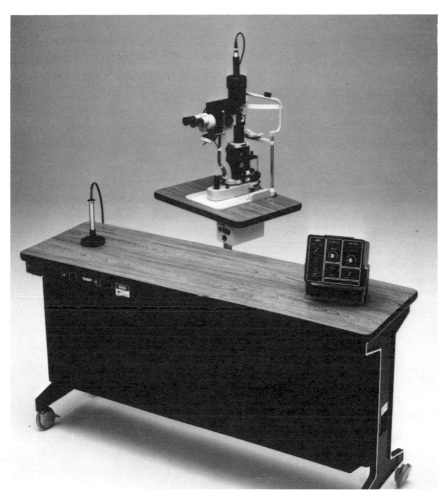

FIGURE 2.1 Argon laser with slit lamp for ophthalmology

488 and 514 nm. Light at these wavelengths will pass through clear and colourless structures without absorption, and without causing thermal damage, and is absorbed by tissues which have its complementary colour red and there is significant absorption by haemoglobin.

This laser was first used in ophthalmology to treat diabetic retinopathy through, and without damage to, the clear anterior parts of the eye. The main role of this laser is to perform photocoagulation of both normal and abnormal blood vessels and some work has been carried out using this laser at higher energy levels to perform slow and relatively imprecise thermal tissue destruction.

The argon laser is used in gastroenterology via a flexible fibre optic endoscope to coagulate bleeding vessels in upper gastrointestinal ulcers, and in a number of controlled studies, control of haemorrhage, a reduction in rate of re-bleeding and reduced mortality have been achieved. In neurosurgery it is used to control both normal and abnormal blood vessels but at present much of the work on the treatment of arteriovenous malformations and aneurysms is experimental. The role of the argon laser via a fine flexible fibre to disobliterate obstructed blood vessels is being researched.

In the treatment of tumours of the tracheobronchial tree and oesophagus using flexible fibre optic instruments, most of the work has been carried out with the neodymium YAG laser. Slow and relatively imprecise tissue destruction can be performed with the argon laser, but it is now only regularly used to 'gut' small tumours which are inaccessible to the carbon dioxide laser, and too close to vital areas for the use of the deeply absorbed neodymium YAG laser.

A number of machines are now available, and in all the argon laser energy is transmitted via a flexible fibre and is aimed by the attenuated beam. Early machines were water-cooled and needed to be plumbed in, providing a fixed and inflexible installation. However, some of the more modern machines are air-cooled and are much more flexible (Figure 2.2) and it appears that there are no significant problems with overheating if the machine is used at high power levels for long periods of time. Argon laser powers of 5–20 watts are available and for ophthalmology, dermatology, neurosurgery and cardiovascular work, a 5 watt tube appears to be adequate, but for control of upper gastrointestinal bleeding and for the removal of tissue, the much more expensive 20 watt laser is needed.

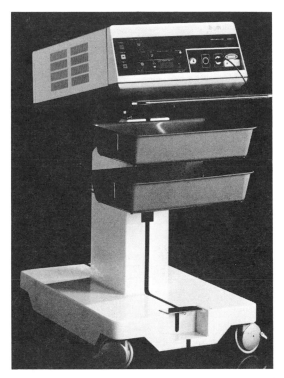

FIGURE 2.2 Argon/krypton laser

Carbon dioxide

The carbon dioxide laser (Figure 2.3a,b) is a 'high-precision, blood-less, light scalpel'. The infrared beam at 10 600 nm wavelength is absorbed by water and tissue destruction is by instantaneous vapor-ization at the relatively low temperature of 100°C. As tissues conduct heat poorly, there is little spread of heat to normal tissues adjacent to the laser wound and, as a result, healing is not complicated by oedema and is rapid and remarkably pain-free.

Much work with this laser is carried out under magnification, using either the operating microscope or colposcope, and the beam is transmitted via a hollow, articulated arm with mirrors at the ar-ticulations. The machines incorporate a low-powered, visible, helium

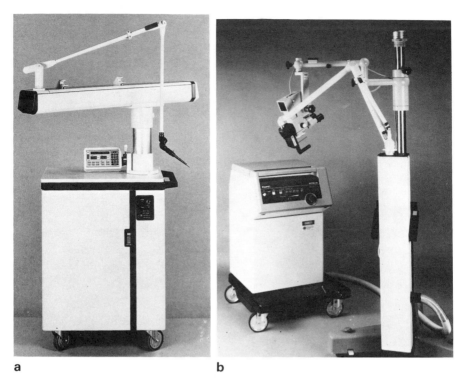

a   b

FIGURE 2.3 (**a**) Carbon dioxide laser with handpiece; (**b**) carbon dioxide laser mounted on microscope

neon laser aiming beam to define the beam path and target area, and this is controlled by a micro-manipulator on the laser delivery head.

The amount of tissue destruction can be controlled with precision by choosing an appropriate power level of the beam and exposure time of the beam on the tissues. There is evidence that a short, sharp dissection technique using high power and short exposure may result in even less damage to adjacent, normal tissues and the recent introduction of pulsed carbon dioxide lasers may prove to be of significant advantage in this area.

The carbon dioxide beam may be used to remove tissue in one of two ways. First, after biopsy, the lesion may be vaporized until a bed of healthy tissue is reached. The second and better technique is to use the beam as a scalpel to excise a lesion with appropriate margins. With this technique the defect is more precisely cut and is no bigger than after vaporization, and the whole lesion is available for histology.

The beam seals blood vessels of up to 0.5 mm in diameter and if the beam is defocused, larger vessels may be controlled. The beam also seals lymphatics, possibly reducing the spread of tumour cells by this route, and seals nerve endings; there is no incidence of neuroma formation.

The main uses of this laser are in ENT and gynaecology. In ENT the laser is used to remove laryngeal lesions with precision, haemostasis and no postoperative oedema and lesions of the mouth and tongue with much reduced morbidity. In gynaecology it is now the 'treatment of choice' for the local destruction of appropriate cervical intraephithelial neoplasia lesions. A large number of patients can tolerate this treatment without anaesthetic, postoperative morbidity and complications are low, and long-term results appear to be excellent.

The carbon dioxide laser provides true 'no-touch' surgery, and is used increasingly in neurosurgery for the precise atraumatic removal of tissue and for the creation of precise lesions for the control of pain.

At low energy levels this laser is being investigated for tissue welding and microvascular anastomosis.

Neodymium YAG

This laser produces infrared coherent light at 1060 nm wavelength, which is deeply absorbed in the tissues without colour or tissue specificity. Its deep absorption means that there is a significant risk of spread of the laser energy to adjacent tissues, even beyond the organ being treated.

The energy of this laser can be transmitted via a flexible fibre and a low-powered, visible helium neon laser is used as the aiming beam. It is used to perform slow but adequate thermal tissue destruction for the removal of tumours in the tracheobronchial tree, oesophagus and bladder. In the removal of tumour tissue there are three distinct layers of damage: first, an area which is vaporized; second, a layer of tissue in which the cells are killed and will slough; and third, a layer of tissue in which the cells are killed but are replaced by fibrous

45

tissue without loss of physical integrity. This third layer of damage means that in the treatment of tumour which involves the whole thickness of the wall of a viscus, there is little risk of perforation. Much of the work on tracheal, bronchial and oesophageal tumours has been for palliation of untreatable disease, but bladder tumours have been treated for cure.

This laser is also used via a flexible fibre optic gastroscope to control bleeding from upper gastrointestinal ulcers and to reduce the incidence of re-bleeding and hence improve survival figures. In controlled series these aims have been achieved, and it has been suggested that this laser is better than the argon laser in this field. The energy is absorbed in tissues around the bleeding vessel, causing damage and fibrosis enabling larger vessels to be controlled than is possible with the argon laser.

The pulsed neodymium YAG laser is being evaluated in ophthalmology for the removal of opaque bodies from within the eye. Short, nanosecond pulses of energy are used, and these create microlesions in which the temperature is raised to more than the temperature of the sun. Using longer pulses of energy the pulsed neodymium YAG laser is being evaluated for the fragmentation of gallstones and renal calculi by photoacoustic effects.

Dye laser

A rhodamine dye is most commonly used in this laser, and it is excited by an argon laser. The dye laser is different from other lasers in that its wavelength can be tuned over a significant range of the visible spectrum. Its energy, which is at best 25% of that of the exciting argon laser, can be transmitted via a flexible fibre and it is aimed by an attenuated beam.

This laser has two main areas of use at present: first, it is used to activate haemotoporphyrin derivative in malignant tumours for the treatment of many forms of localized malignant disease by photoradiation therapy. Second, it has been suggested that both the pulsed and continuous wave dye lasers may prove to be better than the argon laser for the selective destruction of blood vessels within the skin, and these lasers are being extensively researched in the treatment of the port wine stain with some exciting and encouraging early results.

Metal vapour lasers

Copper vapour

This pulsed laser produces blue/green coherent light at wavelengths similar to those produced by the argon laser, and much higher power levels are available. It is being investigated as an alternative to the argon laser in the treatment of the port wine stain and it is already being used to excite dye lasers.

Gold vapour

This laser (Figure 2.4) produces pulsed red light at 628 nm wavelength, which can be used for the activation of intra-tumour haematoporphyrin derivative for photoradiation therapy. Much higher

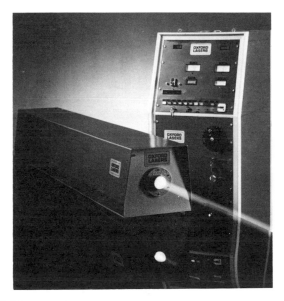

FIGURE 2.4 Gold vapour laser

power levels are produced than are available with the dye laser, and early research suggests that this pulsed laser may prove to be better for tissue penetration and activation of haematoporphyrin derivative than the continuous wave dye laser.

Excimer laser

Excimer lasers are those which utilize, as a lasing medium, substances which only exist in the excited state, such as xenon fluoride. It has been shown that using a xenon fluoride laser emitting at 351 nm it is possible to produce melanosome rupture and necrosis of the basal layer of the epidermis in treated skin. Microscopy shows that the melanosomes rupture in otherwise intact cells, showing that it is possible to damage a particular organelle within a cell.

It has also been shown that it is possible to create extremely precise incisions using excimer lasers, and this may be of great advantage in surgery to the eye and central nervous system.

Ruby

The ruby laser produces pulsed, coherent light at 694 nm, and although much of the early research on the effects of lasers on living tissue was carried out with this laser, it is now only regularly used for the treatment of certain pigmented skin lesions and blue and black tattoos.

Mid lasers

It is somewhat difficult to define a mid laser, as a number of lasers have been used in this context. The helium neon and gallium arsenide lasers are defined as mid lasers, as are the therapeutic lasers, argon, neodymium YAG, and carbon dioxide, when used at less than therapeutic powers. It has been suggested that these lasers can be used to improve wound healing and to relieve pain, but more scientifically acceptable objective evidence from carefully constructed controlled trials is needed before their value is widely accepted.

Cold beam/soft lasers

There was a vogue some years ago for the use of so-called soft or cold beam lasers in the cosmetic industry for treatment of the ageing face by so-called laser face-lifts and laser facial toning. This work continues but there is, as yet, no scientifically acceptable evidence to support the claims made by the manufacturers for their value in this field. It is even difficult to find an acceptable series of photographs taken before and after treatment. Until objective evidence becomes available the case for their use must be considered to be 'not proven'.

SAFETY

Lasers are dangerous as their use in the 'Star Wars' scene testifies! However, although most medical lasers are less powerful than many used in science and industry, all those used therapeutically are in the highest power class – Class IV – and their use 'requires extreme caution'.

The general public and medical profession are well aware of these potential dangers and it must be shown, beyond reasonable doubt, that safe lasers are being used in a safe manner by fully trained personnel on appropriate clinical conditions. It is, happily, relatively easy to conform with the first conditions but the subject of training in laser techniques and safety, and the qualifications to practise laser surgery, remain the subject of debate which, on occasions, becomes heated.

The machine

Each country has safety codes which cover the electrical and laser safety of medical lasers and their installation, and it is up to the practitioner to check with the supplier that his machine conforms to all the appropriate regulations and that it has been installed safely.

Safety codes and safe use

In the UK the safe use of lasers is controlled by the British Standards Code BS4803, the Health and Safety at Work and the Factories Acts, and the 'Guidance on the Safe Use of Lasers in Medical Practice', recently produced by the DHSS. It would obviously be inappropriate to detail all the regulations in this chapter but mention must be made of some of the most important ones.

First, all codes insist on the appointment of a local laser safety officer[1] who will be responsible for all aspects of laser safety and who will produce codes of safe practice for each laser in each clinical situation.

The main risk from lasers is damage to the eyes of a patient or a member of the operating theatre personnel, and the site of damage depends on the wavelength of the laser. The carbon dioxide laser would cause a corneal burn whereas the visible lasers cause retinal damage.

It is, of course, extremely unlikely that anyone would be injured by the direct beam, but an injury could be caused if the beam were reflected back into the operating theatre from an instrument or retractor.

The eyes of the patient must be protected by appropriate, carefully fixed eye covers (Figure 2.5). If a slit lamp, operating microscope or endoscope is being used, the eyes of the surgeon are protected by either the optics of the microscope in the case of the carbon dioxide laser, a shutter with the argon laser, or filters with the neodymium YAG laser. However, for all other usage, appropriate eye-wear must be worn. All the codes of practice insist that fully laser-proof eye-wear, appropriate to the laser being used, is provided for all those in the operating theatre, and the specifications of the various forms of eye protection are clearly defined.

A hazard almost unique to otolaryngology is that of anaesthetic tube combustion. If an anaesthetic tube made of combustible material and carrying anaesthetic gases is struck by the carbon dioxide laser beam it will ignite, and a number of serious accidents have been reported. This hazard must be slight in the dermatological use of the lasers but it might be relevant in the treatment of lesions around the mouth under general anaesthetic. However, the tube can

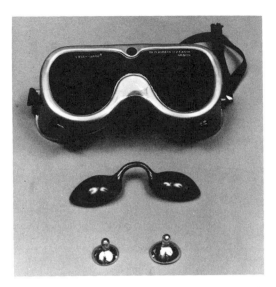

FIGURE 2.5 Eye protection for use with argon laser – goggles, shield, contact lenses

readily be protected by wrapping it in aluminium foil or by covering it with a thick, moist swab.

Government controls

Recent government legislation insists that all premises in which lasers are used must be inspected and certified.

Training programmes

Despite controls of the machine, its safe use and the premises on which it is used, there are at present no regulations to control the use of lasers by medical and surgical practitioners. It is obviously essential that all those who use lasers have a working knowledge of laser physics and laser/tissue interaction, and a thorough knowledge of laser techniques in their particular discipline and all aspects of laser safety. A number of cases of laser malpractice have been widely reported in the media and have seriously damaged the image of medical lasers. It is to be hoped that some official policies will be formulated to prevent the use of lasers by untrained medical personnel.

THE PORT WINE STAIN

Introduction

The argon laser is, at present, the treatment of choice for the hitherto untreatable port wine stain, and this condition must represent the single most important indication for laser therapy in dermatology. Recent research suggests that the tuneable dye laser, both pulsed and continuous wave, may prove to be superior to the argon laser in the selective destruction of dermal blood vessels. However, despite some exciting early results, it will be several years before it will be shown if this laser can produce superior clinical results, and the argon laser will be in use in this field for many more years. Much work is in progress to define an optimal treatment technique to give the best clinical results with the lowest incidence of scarring. An editorial in the *Lancet* in 1981[2] described the argon laser as 'a new ray of hope for port wine stains' and already some excellent results are being obtained with a wide range of treatment techniques.

Incidence

A persistent port wine stain is thought to occur in between 0.1 and 0.5% of the population. They do not appear to be genetically determined and no aetiological factors have been identified. The lesion often occurs on the face in the distribution of the fifth (trigeminal) cranial nerve, and if it involves the ophthalmic and/or the maxillary division, 45% of the patients will have incipient or actual glaucoma and 1–2% intracranial involvement with the Sturge–Weber syndrome.

Histology

A port wine stain is composed of a network of abnormal capillaries in the outer dermis – there appears to be both an increase in the number and in the dilatation of these vessels. The overlying epidermis is essentially normal and the colour of the blood in the capillaries shows through the epidermis, giving the port wine stain its characteristic pink, red or purple colour. A number of histological types have been described and Ohmori and Huang[3] refer to the constricted, dilated, intermediate and deep located lesions, and they correlate the histological type with its response to argon laser therapy. Noe *et al.*[4] have studied the histology of the port wine stain in detail, in an attempt to predict accurately those which will respond well, and have shown that a good response could be expected in those lesions in which more than 5% of the dermis was occupied by blood vessels, the mean vessel area was greater than $2500\,\mu m^2$, and the proportion of vessels containing erythrocytes was greater than 15%. They refer to the haemoglobin target of each birth mark.

Previous treatment techniques

In the past a wide range of treatment techniques had been used but none gave consistently satisfactory results and the port wine stain remained essentially untreatable. Treatments used included thorium X, radioactive phosphorus, dermabrasion, cryotherapy, excision and grafting and over-tattooing of the lesion with opaque pigments. However, a majority of patients were left untreated and were told that no specific treatment was available apart from the use of camouflage make-up. Despite an increase in the availability of make-up and improved quality, it has been estimated that not more than 30% of patients wear it regularly. For obvious reasons it is much more difficult for a man to wear heavy make-up than a woman. However, if a patient does regularly use camouflage make-up he or she may be unwilling to be seen in public without it, and clinic staff must be aware of this problem and must attempt to keep the patient out of the public eye while in the clinic.

Psychology

Patients with a port wine stain feel marked out as being different, and failures in life are blamed on the birth mark. Patients often blame the parents, and the parents often feel guilty, believing that some unwise act during pregnancy has resulted in the port wine stain on their child. A port wine stain almost invariably has a devastating effect on the life of an individual and the effect cannot be directly quantified with the size or colour of the mark. A significant number of patients threaten, and a very small number of patients commit, suicide. Despite some protestations to the contrary almost all patients wish to be relieved of this birthmark at any age, but are somewhat unrealistically perfectionist in their expectation of the results of treatment. When told that the mark may not disappear, but will show marked lightening with the preservation of skin texture, they often experience disappointment. However, when the test patch is performed and when they can see the mark lightening with treatment their mood almost invariably changes and many appear very delighted with a result which could not objectively be described as excellent or perfect.

The aim of therapy must be to treat a patient at as early an age as possible, and sadly it appears, at present, that treatment in the young is less satisfactory than those above the age of 17. However, with further research it may be possible using the argon or the dye laser to treat children below the age of 10.

Treatment of a port wine stain with the argon laser (Figures 2.6–2.8)

White Caucasian epidermis transmits argon laser energy with minimal absorption and suffers minimal thermal damage. There is some slight injury, however, but no irreversible damage to the secondary skin appendages and after treatment the epidermis should return to normal or show minimal atrophic changes. If the epidermis is pigmented, either racially or by a heavy sun tan, treatment is less satisfactory as there is significant absorption of the argon laser energy in the pigment in the basal layer of the epidermis with greater epidermal damage giving an increased risk of scarring; also

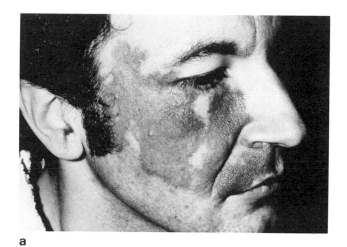

a

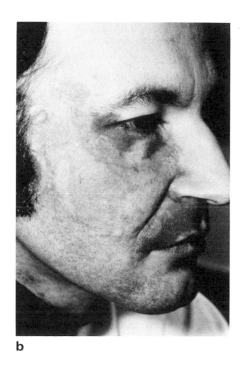

b

FIGURE 2.6 (**a**) Port-wine stain before treatment with argon laser; (**b**) after treatment with argon laser – eyelid and upper lip not yet treated

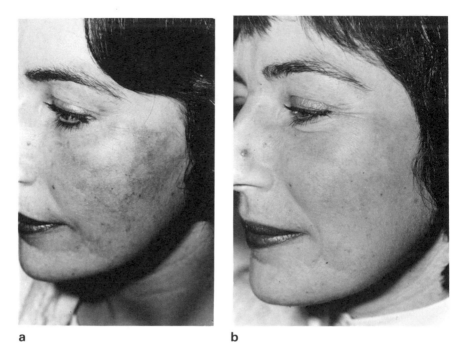

a   b

FIGURE 2.7 (**a**) Port-wine stain before treatment with argon laser; (**b**) after treatment

the capillaries of a port wine stain are protected from the laser energy.

Having been transmitted through the epidermis, the beam is absorbed by the blood in the capillaries and also by the endothelium causing thermal damage and thrombosis. It has been shown by Apfelberg *et al.*[5] that over a period of months the thrombosed 'vessel layer' is replaced by colourless fibrous tissue with a marked reduction in the number of vessels, and with others being reduced to narrow slits. This results in a significant reduction in the colour of the mark with a preservation of normal skin texture. It has also been shown that these results are stable for at least 7 years, and there are no pathological grounds for expecting a relapse after this time.

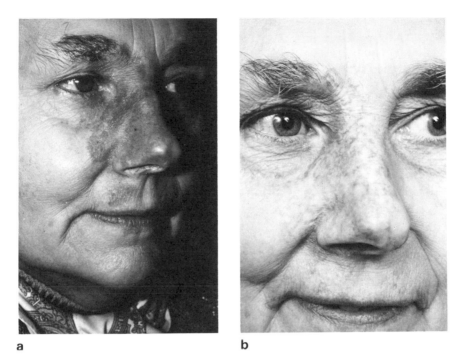

a   b

FIGURE 2.8 (a) Port-wine stain before treatment with argon laser; (b) after treatment

Treatment technique

A very wide range of treatment techniques have been described in the literature [6–8], and all seem to achieve a similar number of good/excellent results. However, the incidence of scarring varies very considerably within the reported series, and the incidence of both atrophic and hypertrophic scarring seems to be directly related to the total energy delivered. As with all surgical and medical procedures, the classical rule must apply – 'Make the patient better if you can, but whatever you do don't make him worse.' If significant hypertrophic or atrophic scarring is produced the deformity will have been made worse, and it will be much more difficult to conceal with make-up. To achieve the optimal results with the lowest incidence of scarring a large number of workers now adopt a 'low-power' technique.

Prediction of a good response

It appears that dark, purple marks respond better than light, pink ones, and as there is a tendency for marks to darken with age, results will tend to be better in older patients. There is evidence to show that a good result can be expected in patients over the age of 17 but below that age, and in particular below the age of 10, results are less predictable.

However, more evidence is needed before authoritative comments can be made on the youngest age at which treatment can be success-fully performed. A study of many of the reported series shows that very few children have been treated, and this is partly due to the fact that almost all of the work has been carried out under local anaes-thetic and it is very difficult, if not impossible, to treat a facial mark in a child in this way. Research is in progress in several centres on the treatment of children, where necessary under general anaesthetic, to determine the youngest age at which treatment can be carried out, and some encouraging results are being obtained with no significant incidence of scarring.

Marks on the face appear to respond better than those on the limbs or trunk. However, this may not represent a difference in skin response, but may be due to the very large area of skin occupied by a mark on the trunk or a limb which makes treatment technically very difficult and extremely time-consuming.

From the histological studies described above, it can be seen that certain histological types respond well, but Ohmori and Huang[3] have shown that, using a spectrophotometer, there is a very close corre-lation between the colour of a mark and its histological type.

Many consider that it is inappropriate to biopsy these benign lesions in all cases to aid prediction, and the non-invasive technique of transcutaneous microscopy is being evaluated[9]. With this tech-nique the vascular patterns of a port wine stain can be studied *in vivo*, and a number of different vascular patterns can be identified. It will be possible to classify port wine stains, and it is hoped that this classification will aid accurate prediction. It is also possible to follow treatment at all stages with this technique.

Consultation

At the first consultation before a test patch is performed, the patient must be given full details of the treatment with a realistic percentage chance of success and of scarring. After an opportunity to ask questions the patient will be in a position to sign an appropriately informed consent form.

Test patch

Despite the relative wealth of predicting features of a port wine stain, some which should respond well do not and vice-versa, and many workers carry out a test patch to assess the response of an individual's birthmark to argon laser therapy. The test patch is performed under local anaesthetic without adrenalin, which is deeply injected beneath the area of the mark to be tested.

Some workers use a constant power level for the test patch and for the subsequent treatment, if the test is successful, but others determine the appropriate power for each patient. In the Southampton Laser Unit the 'minimal blanching power technique'[10] was developed to ensure that treatment is carried out at the lowest possible effective power to reduce scarring to a minimum. Using this technique the incidence of scarring is below the previously best reported figure of 2%.

For the test an automatically repeated pluse of 0.2 s duration is used. The spot size of 1 mm is kept constant by a spacer fitted to the handpiece described by the author in 1982[11]. Starting at a power of 0.2 watts, well below the lowest recorded blanching power, the power is increased in increments of 0.2 watt until blanching of the lesion is achieved. Using this technique almost all patients will need between 0.6 and 1.0 watts for clinical blanching. The beam is then used to erase an area of the mark of about 1 cm² in an inconspicuous site.

The epidermis is not entirely transparent to the argon laser light and suffers some slight damage, and the tested area weeps for a few days. A light scab forms which separates after about 10–14 days, leaving the treated area red. This colour fades for up to 15 months after treatment, but the test patch is usually assessed after 4–6 months, when one of three results will be found:

1. good,
2. inadequate blanching,
3. scar (atrophic or hypertrophic).

Good response

The test area will show complete or very satisfactory blanching with a preservation of normal skin texture. If a good result is obtained then the lesion will be treated under either local or general anaesthetic.

Inadequate blanching

If the test area shows too much residual colour a second test patch will be performed using a higher power of 0.2 watts above the minimal blanching power, and this sequence will be repeated at intervals of 4–6 months until a satisfactory test patch is achieved, or scarring develops. If the minimal blanching power technique is used a second test patch will be needed in about 20% of patients.

Scarring

With this technique the incidence of either atrophic or hypertrophic scarring should be less than 2%, but if it occurs in an adult the patient may not be treatable. However, having tested more than 250 patients only two adults have shown slight hypertrophic scarring in the test patch and both had developed hypertrophic changes in abdominal wounds previously.

If scarring occurs in a child then a further test will be carried out after a period of years, but to date only mild atrophic changes have been observed in a small number of children.

Treatment technique

Programme

In the Southampton Laser Unit, at the time of consultation, a test patch is performed which is assessed after 6 months, when a treatment will be carried out if the test patch is satisfactory. The result of the first treatment will be assessed after 3–4 months to ensure that there are no unexpected adverse reactions when a larger area has been treated. However, if the area is satisfactory then the whole lesion will be treated in a number of sessions depending on the size of the lesion under local or general anaesthetic at intervals of 6–8 weeks.

Treatment itself is tedious and time-consuming, and the whole treatment programme for a patient may take many months or even years. All the work in the Southampton Laser Unit is carried out under the National Health Service, and it has been said by those in the private sector that this type of programme is not commercially viable.

Power density

A wide range of treatment powers have been recorded in the literature but a measurement of power alone is meaningless as the power density of treatment (watts/cm^2) is the relevant measurement. The power density depends on the output power of the laser and the area of the laser imprint and, with many of the free hand techniques, the area of the spot changes constantly with the focused beam at a slightly different angle to, and distance from, the skin. To avoid this constant variation in power density a spacer on the handpiece should be used to keep the spot in focus and the beam at right angles to the skin.

Exposure

A significant range of exposures has been described in the literature, but much of the reported work has been carried out with an automatically repeated pulse of 0.2 s which appears to be a 'comfortable' exposure to use with the free hand technique. However, recently, a considerable number of treatments have been carried out using a 'continuous exposure' and the beam is used with an 'air brush' technique to erase the mark. It is of course essential to move the beam at a constant speed over the skin. In theory there could be an increased risk of scarring as more energy is delivered to the skin. However, test patches performed with a continuous exposure technique have been carefully compared with patches performed with an intermittent exposure and no significant differences have been observed – the clinical blanching appears to be more uniform. The continuous exposure technique is far less tedious and time-consuming and even using a 1 mm diameter spot, birth mark erasure is relatively rapid and easy.

Erasure technique

Apfelberg and others described the 'zebra stripe' technique in which untreated 5 mm stripes were left between similar treated stripes to improve epidermal regeneration. However, in a subsequent paper in 1983[12] they found that there was residual evidence of striping in a significant number of cases, and they concluded that 'no definite benefit can be attributed to the zebra stripe technique'.

Most workers simply use the laser to obtain clinical blanching but debate continues as to whether the laser imprints should touch or should overlap, and techniques using both have been described. If the beam is used to create clinical blanching, there will be some 'inevitable' overlap and in the Southampton Unit, where the actual area treated, as measured by the number of laser impacts multiplied by the area of each imprint was calculated, it was found to be 1.5 times the area of treatment. If the continuous exposure technique is used, then this problem is obviously not relevant.

Whichever erasure technique is used the beam must be moved along and not across natural skin lines and long, straight lines must be avoided. Particular care must be taken in the erasure of marks on the eyelids and on the lips, where, in all series, the incidence of scarring is highest. It appears appropriate to perform separate test patches on the lips, and in a number of cases a lower power will be needed to create blanching of a lesion on the lip than on the cheek.

Results

A wide range of treatment techniques have been used and a range of different criteria for the grading of results. However, in most series in patients with a good prognosis – an older patient with a dark facial mark – a satisfactory result can be obtained in 60–80% of cases. After argon laser therapy the treated area often shows a transient post-traumatic hyperpigmentation and the end result may leave some permanent hypopigmentation. Results in younger patients are less predicatable, but a study of birth marks using transcutaneous microscopy shows that a number of young patients have 'old' birth marks and careful studies will show which patients can be treated at an early age.

Another change in the birth mark which tends to occur with age is the development of a nodular texture to the skin. If the 'nodules' are treated, often at a higher power, they can be destroyed with a marked improvement in the texture of the skin after treatment.

Cooling of lesions

Gilchrest *et al.*[13] were able to improve results by chilling the skin before treatment, and found significantly better test patches and final results than in unchilled cases.

Retreatment

It has been shown by Cosman[14] that if a low-powered treatment technique has been used, then retreatment may be carried out after a period of 15–18 months with further cosmetic improvement and with a chance of scarring no higher than after the original treatment.

Conclusions

It is imperative to record all treatment parameters accurately so that techniques and results can be compared. It must be hoped that an optimal treatment technique or optimal techniques for marks of various types, in patients of various ages, will be developed to produce the best results with the lowest possible incidence of scarring.

Already a wide range of techniques are producing satisfactory results in a majority of patients with this hitherto untreatable condition, and with further research results in older patients must improve and it should be possible to treat patients at a much younger age.

Treatment of a port wine stain with a dye laser

Using a tuneable dye laser with a rhodamine dye at 577 nm, Greenwald et al.[15] compared its effects on blood vessels in the skin with the effects of the argon laser. They found that the dye laser caused much more selective damage to the cutaneous vascular plexus than the argon laser and at much lower energy levels. Using a continuous wave dye laser at 540 nm, Hulsbergen-Henning and van Gemert[16] treated three patients and compared the test patches with patches produced with an argon laser. They too found that the dye laser produced much more selective vessel damage and the end result after 5 months appeared to be 'normal skin'.

A considerable amount of research is in progress using both continuous wave and pulsed dye lasers to treat port wine stains. The results of these trials will show if the dye laser can produce superior results to those which can be obtained with the argon laser.

Treatment of a port wine stain with the carbon dioxide laser

It has been suggested by Ratz et al.[17] that certain port wine stains can be treated by the carbon dioxide laser, particularly pale, pink ones which are least suitable for argon laser therapy. However, with the water-absorbed carbon dioxide laser the epidermis must be vaporized before the abnormal capillary network is reached, and the technique must represent a precise form of laser dermabrasion. As such, the risk of scarring must be significant. With this technique the skin is removed layer by layer down to the capillary network and this is vaporized until no further vessels can be identified. Re-epithelialization occurs after 4–6 weeks and only 9% of patients developed hypertrophic scarring with excellent results in 57% of patients.

A small number of patients have been treated with this technique to date and it is too early to state whether the carbon dioxide laser will be of value in the treatment of port wine stains.

Treatment of a port wine stain with the neodymium YAG laser

A small number of patients have been treated using this laser with the skin surface cooled by water, and a number of satisfactory results have been obtained. However, it has been stated that the chance of scarring is greater than with the argon laser and more work is needed to show the value of this laser in the treatment of the port wine stain.

OTHER VASCULAR LESIONS

Spider naevi

The argon laser can be used to treat these lesions and an intermittent pulse of 0.2 s of about 1 W is aimed at the 'body' of the spider until, after a few impacts, the spider 'dies'!

Telangiectasia

The superficial vessels are treated similarly to a port wine stain and some very satisfactory results can be obtained.

Hereditary haemorrhagic telangiectasia

It is possible to destroy the lesions of this condition using either the carbon dioxide or argon laser with excellent results, but there is, as with any technique, a tendency for these lesions to recur in other sites.

Leg veins

It was hoped that leashes of small leg vessels associated with varicose veins would be suitable for treatment with the argon laser. Unfortunately results appear to be rather unpredictable and certainly less good than had been hoped. If these vessels are to be treated a test patch should be performed to assess their response to argon laser therapy.

Strawberry naevus

These lesions regress with age and therefore treatment should be avoided if possible. However, it has been shown that these lesions will respond to argon laser therapy and in exceptional circumstances treatment may be carried out.

Rhinophyma

The excessive tissue can be ablated by either the argon or carbon dioxide lasers and allowed to heal with satisfactory cosmetic results.

Tuberous sclerosis

The fibroangiomas described traditionally as adenomata sebaceum will respond to ablation with the argon laser and a marked cosmetic improvement can be obtained. However, a majority of patients are, unfortunately, unable to appreciate this cosmetic improvement and relatively few patients are suitable for treatment.

SKIN SURGERY WITH THE CARBON DIOXIDE LASER

Introduction

A considerable amount of skin surgery is performed by the carbon dioxide laser and has been described in the literature[18]. Undoubtedly it is possible to perform a wide range of procedures with this laser, but as stated earlier, a laser should only be used when it can perform a specific task better than established, conventional techniques, and in many of the techniques described in the literature it is difficult to identify these advantages. Certainly for many of the indications the advantages are too slight to justify the expense of purchasing a laser.

A number of machines have been set up in clinics within the private sector and although some reputable surgery is being performed these machines have been responsible for the well-publicized cases of laser abuse which have resulted in at least two practitioners being struck off the medical register. This abuse has significantly damaged the valid use of lasers in medicine and surgery.

There is an enormous demand for 'cosmetic' skin surgery and in this field, beyond all others, it must be clearly shown why lasers should be used, not just that they can be used to perform particular procedures.

Incisions

It is possible to cut skin incisions with the carbon dioxide laser using a handpiece but it has been shown from the very earliest research with this laser by Hall[19], that incisions are no quicker to cut, and that they heal more slowly with no better scar than incisions cut by scalpel.

It is possibly an advantage to cut incisions with the carbon dioxide laser in patients with a haemorrhagic tendency, as the sealing of small blood vessels will provide better haemostasis, but these cases are uncommon. It is also possible to cut vascular tissues with this laser but major vessels cannot be controlled.

Dissection

In dissection the 'no-touch' surgery is a positive disadvantage as the lack of proprioceptive feedback from fingers or instruments makes the dissection of tissue planes much more difficult.

Burns

It has been shown by Fidler[20] that it is possible to deslough burns, to prepare them for skin grafting, with the carbon dioxide laser with a significant reduction in blood loss. However, the procedure may be slower than with the scalpel which, in children, may allow greater heat loss.

Infected ulcers

Infected ulcers may be prepared for skin grafting with the carbon dioxide laser, which is used to remove infected debris and to sterilize the base.

Mohs' surgery

It has been shown by Bailin *et al.*[21] that Mohs' surgery can be performed by carbon dioxide laser. In this technique a malignant lesion is removed 'layer by layer' and each section removed in this way is entirely suitable for histological assessment by frozen section. The removal is continued until a bed of healthy tissue is reached, and this bed is suitable for skin grafting.

Warts and condylomata acuminata

The carbon dioxide laser is of undoubted advantage in the rapid removal of multiple lesions such as warts and condylomata acuminata. Under local or occasionally general anaesthetic these lesions can be quickly vaporized and the wounds remain clean and heal rapidly. In the treatment of condylomata acuminata a large number of series have been reported in the gynaecological literature to show the benefits of this laser in the ease of treatment and in the low incidence of recurrence.

Malignant lesions

All forms of malignant lesion of the skin may be excised with the carbon dioxide laser and potential advantages for the use of this laser are the sealing of lymphatics by the beam during surgery and the low level of tissue manipulation, possibly leading to reduced spread of malignant cells. In addition, there is no shock impact when the beam strikes the tissues and therefore no tendency to force malignant cells into adjacent tissues; nor are there any viable cell components in the vapour produced by tissue destruction with the carbon dioxide laser.

However, despite a number of series describing the use of the carbon dioxide laser in this field, there is as yet no evidence from controlled trials to show improved cure rates, and it has been stated that the carbon dioxide laser is less good than the scalpel in the treatment of malignant melanoma.

Keloid

In the treatment of this condition it has been suggested that if the keloid is excised with the carbon dioxide laser, and the base then injected with triamcinolone, the resulting scar may still be prominent but the keloid will not reform.

TREATMENT OF SKIN LESIONS WITH THE NEODYMIUM YAG LASER

The treatment of benign, semi-malignant and malignant skin tumours using the neodymium YAG laser was described by Brunner et al. in 1985[22]. They treated 80 patients with assorted skin lesions, of whom 45 had basal cell carcinoma. The energy from this laser is deeply absorbed in the tissues without colour or tissue specificity. At high energy levels tissue will be vaporized, but at the lower energy levels described in the paper, thermal cell death is produced and the tissue destroyed in this way sloughs over a period of days.

Skin surgery carried out with this laser lacks the precision of the carbon dioxide laser, but it might be of value in the treatment of some vascular lesions. If lesions of a significant area are treated there must be a significant risk of cosmetically unacceptable scarring. Further work will establish the value of this laser in dermatological surgery, but it is hard to see at present how its role in this field could justify the purchase of a machine for this speciality alone.

TATTOOS

As with all medical problems prevention is better than cure, but there does appear to be an increasing interest in the acquisition of tattoos, particularly by the young who are unaware that the tattoo cannot be removed by any technique without leaving some form of scar. Tattoos may be applied either by amateur or professional tattoo artistes. The amateur uses India ink, soot and needles to apply the tattoo, and pigment is deposited widely throughout the layers of the skin and often into the subcutaneous fat. The depth of pigment application by professionals is much more constant, although it may lie deeply in the dermis and some reflective pigments are used which are more difficult to treat with any form of laser.

The pulsed ruby laser is used to treat some blue and black tattoos with excellent results, and some amateur tattoos can be made to disappear. However, much of the work on tattoos has been carried out by the carbon dioxide and argon lasers.

Although colour selective absorption is of critical importance in the treatment of the port wine stain, using the argon laser it does not appear to be significant in the treatment of tattoos. Both lasers are used in essentially the same manner to treat tattoos, but a number of different techniques have been described[23,24]. The lasers are used to remove the skin layer by layer down to the pigment, which is then destroyed and the resulting wound allowed to heal, in the hope that the resulting scar will prove to be more acceptable to the patient than the original tattoo. The use of the operating microscope is described, and some workers remove only part of the pigment at each treatment session, whereas others use a striped technique to improve epidermal regeneration. In the postoperative period pain

70

may be significant, and steroids may be used to reduce the incidence of hypertrophic scarring.

Lasers can be used to perform precise dermabrasion to remove the pigment of tattoos but unfortunately they do not offer the magic remedy for this problem that has been suggested in the media. If used carefully under magnification the scarring produced by the laser removal of tattoos will be minimal and certainly offensive names and symbols can be blurred. The patients must be told exactly what to expect, and a majority will then prefer the scar, which has no stigma, to the stigma of the original tattoo. However, it is unnecessary to state that if an imperfect technique is used, or if lasers fall into the wrong hands, then disasters can occur.

MID-LASERS

There is considerable interest, particularly in Italy, in the use of so-called mid lasers for the treatment of pain in sports injuries and rheumatoid conditions, and for the promotion of wound healing. Several lasers are used in this context: the helium neon producing red light, the infrared gallium arsenide and the argon, neodymium YAG, ruby and carbon dioxide lasers used at low power levels.

One major problem with this use of lasers is that no-one has, as yet, offered any adequate explanation of their mode of action, but all workers state that it is 'non-thermal'.

In the treatment of pain the use of the helium neon and gallium arsenide lasers is escalating, and the majority of results reported in the medical and paramedical literature are anecdotal and uncontrolled. However, some adequately controlled studies have been reported but more are needed before the value of these lasers is widely accepted by the medical profession.

The late Professor Mester from Hungary produced a large number of papers to show the value of mid lasers in the promotion of wound healing, and these papers were reviewed by his son in 1985[25] after his death. However, much of his work was uncontrolled and the results have not been repeatable in other centres. Several controlled wound healing experiments in animals have been performed and reported with no clear evidence to show that the laser-treated wounds healed more rapidly. In one trial, however, reported by Surinchak et al.[26] they found that the strength of the laser treated wound was 55% greater than the control at 14 days, but this difference reduced to 16% at 28 days. It was suggested that this difference might be due to increased fibroblast activity, and a suggestion that laser light affects the activity of these cells is a continuing theme throughout much of the work in this field. There has been little or no objective evidence to support this hypothesis until recently, when two studies were reported at conference showing definite objective evidence of an alteration in the behaviour of fibroblasts exposed to mid laser energy, produced by the helium neon laser. Further studies must be awaited with great interest.

COLD BEAM/SOFT LASERS

It has been suggested that the low-powered so-called cold beam or soft lasers are of value in the treatment of the ageing face by 'laser face-lifts' or 'laser facial toning'. To date no acceptable scientific evidence has been produced to validate these claims and no series of pre- and post-treatment photographs of an acceptable quality has been produced to show the value of the helium neon and gallium arsenide lasers in this field.

At present, although one must keep an open mind, and although the level of 'proof' required in the cosmetic field is rather different from that required in medicine, it must be said that the efficacy of this form of therapy has not yet been established.

PHOTORADIATION THERAPY

Photoradiation therapy (PRT) is a new and exciting approach to the management of malignant disease, and although it cannot be regarded as a 'panacea for all forms of cancer' it does represent an exciting development in the management of many forms of localized malignant disease and appears particularly appropriate for tumours of the skin. It has been said by Kennedy (personal communication), one of the pioneers of the technique, that PRT now represents the 'treatment of choice' for multiple basal cell carcinoma.

The killing of paramoecium sensitized by acridine dye and exposed to light, was noted by Raab[27] at the beginning of this century, and since that time many tumour sensitizers have been and are being investigated. However, only one haematoporphyrin derivative (HPD) has reached a stage where it can be used for clinical trials. Recently the active component of the mixture of porphyrins has been identified as dihaematoporphyrin ether (DHE), but many believe that further work on the identification of the active component is appropriate.

HPD was first produced by Swartz from haematoporphyrin, and was used by Lipson et al.[28] for the identification, and later for the therapy, of malignant tumours.

It has been shown in a number of studies that after an intravenous injection, HPD is widely distributed in the body but is then selectively retained by malignant tissues. The mechanism for this retention remains uncertain but it is thought to be due to the abnormal tumour circulation. However, some recent quantitative fluorescence studies have suggested that, in addition, there may be an increased take-up of HPD by malignant tissues.

When exposed to blue/violet light, tumour containing HPD will fluoresce, and a close correlation has been found between fluorescence and a malignant histology. Some very exciting work has been carried out using this tumour fluorescence in the diagnosis of early bronchial carcinoma using a fluorescent bronchoscopic technique in which a krypton laser is used as the light source, and an image intensifier to identify the areas of fluorescence. The fluorescence has also been used to identify malignant areas in multi-focal disease of the bladder.

When tumour containing HPD is exposed to red light it has been shown that singlet oxygen is produced by energy transfer from the excited prophyrin molecule and this highly reactive, transient state of the oxygen molecule is cytotoxic by oxidizing sensitive bonds.

In the development of this technique a number of both filtered and unfiltered light sources were used, but it became apparent that the argon pumped dye laser was the best source of the monochromatic red light needed for PRT at a wavelength of 630 nm which could be transmitted via a flexible fibre. HPD is better activated by blue/green light but this does not penetrate adequately into the tissues and 630 nm is the optimal wavelength for tissue penetration and HPD activation. Recently, pulsed red light at 628 nm produced by the gold vapour laser has been used in PRT. This laser can produce much higher power levels, appears more stable than the majority of dye laser systems, and it has been suggested that the pulsed light is better for tissue penetration and HPD activation than the light produced by the continuous wave dye laser.

Although the technique of photoradiation therapy has been discussed in various national and international medical meetings, it has come to be identified with a number of laser societies, and discussion of the technique appears appropriate in this chapter.

A number of *in vitro* studies have been performed and it has also been shown that PRT can ablate both induced and naturally occurring tumours in animals. Several clinical trials have been performed and more are in progress on bronchial carcinoma for the palliation of advanced disease and for cure in a small number of inoperable early cases, for bladder tumours and tumours of the head and neck, eye, brain, oesophagus and both primary and secondary skin tumours.

Protocols for treatment have been established and all are essentially similar.

On day one the patient is given HPD intravenously in a dose of 3 mg/kg body weight, and no serious side-effects have been reported from the injection. DHE is given in a dose of 1.5-2 mm/kg. All patients develop significant skin photosensitization which lasts for 3-4 weeks, and many patients find this very inconvenient. Patients are advised to stay out of direct light for this time, and some help can be obtained from sun block creams.

Three days later, when HPD is distributed in the optimal tumour/ normal tissue ratio, the tumour is photoirradiated. For many tumours surface irradiation is performed using a straight cut fibre or one with a micro-lens at the tip, to give a more straight-sided beam. Fibres with a diffusing cylinder tip are used to treat circumferential lesions of the bronchus or oesophagus and these can be implanted into large tumours. For the treatment of the inside of a hollow viscus a tip with a diffusing bulb end may be used.

The delivery power will depend on the power of the laser and the area to be treated, and it has been suggested that a minimal treatment power of $15\,mW/cm^2$ may be needed.

For ulcerated tumours a total dose of $100-200$ Joules/cm² is needed to create maximal tumour necrosis which, with surface irradiation, will be to a depth of about 1 cm. For subcutaneous nodules of the chest wall from breast carcinoma, a total dose of 25 Joules/cm² will destroy the tumour with preservation of the overlying skin.

As mentioned already, Kennedy from Ontario has suggested that for multiple basal cell carcinoma, PRT is now the treatment of choice, but the majority of work on skin lesions has been in the treatment of multi-nodular metastatic disease of the chest wall from breast carcinoma. Dr Thomas J. Dougherty of Roswell Park Memorial Institute, Buffalo, who has pioneered much of this work, has estimated that a complete response to treatment in this disease can be obtained in 60-80% of patients (unpublished).

An advantage of this form of treatment is that it can be repeated as often as necessary and does not appear to interfere with other modalities of treatment for malignant disease. One pilot study has been carried out in Britain to date and reported by Carruth and McKenzie[29].

When this technique has been fully evaluated by carefully designed clinical trials, it must play an important part in the management of many forms of localised, malignant disease and it appears particularly appropriate for the management of many forms of skin tumour.

CONCLUSIONS

When used appropriately, lasers can offer advantages to both surgeon and patient which are unique to this modality. However, when lasers are used inappropriately, or fall into the wrong hands, disasters can occur and every attempt must be made to ensure that lasers are only used by fully trained medical personnel in a totally safe manner, on appropriate clinical conditions.

References

1. Carruth, J. A. S. and McKenzie, A. L. (1982). The argon laser in dermatology: safety aspects. *Clin. Exp. Dermatol.*, **7**, 244-5
2. Editorial (1981). New ray of hope for port wine stains. *Lancet*, **1**, 480
3. Ohmori, S. and Huang, C.-K. (1981). Recent progress in the treatment of port wine staining by argon laser: some observations on the prognostic value of relative spectro-reflectance (RSR) and the histological classification of lesions. *Br. J. Plast. Surg.*, **34**, 249-57
4. Noe, J. M., Berksy, S. H., Geer, D. E. and Rosen, S. (1980), Port wine stains and response to argon laser therapy: successful treatment and the predicative role of colour, age and biopsy. *Plast. Reconstr. Surg.*, **65**(2), 130-6
5. Apfelberg, D. B., Kosek, J., Maser, M. R. and Lash, H. (1979). Histology of port wine stains following argon laser treatment. *Br. J. Plast. Surg.*, **32**, 232-7
6. Apfelberg, D. B., Maser, M. R., Lash, H. and Rivera, J. L. (1980). Progress report on extended clinical use of the argon laser for cutaneous lesions. *Lasers Surg. Med.*, **1**, 71-83
7. Cosman, B. (1980). Clinical experience in the laser therapy of port wine stains. *Lasers Surg. Med.*, **1**, 133-52
8. Touquet, V. L. R. and Carruth, J. A. S. (1984). Review of the treatment of port wine stains with the argon laser. *Lasers Surg. Med.*, **4**, 191-9
9. Shakespeare, P. and Carruth, J. A. S. (1985). Evaluation of a port wine stain by transcutaneous microscopy. *Lasers Med. Sci.*, (In press)
10. Carruth, J. A. S. (1984). Argon laser in the treatment of port wine stains. *J. R. Soc. Med.* **77**, 722
11. Carruth, J. A. S. (1982). The establishment of precise physical parameters for the treatment of the port wine stain with the argon laser. *Lasers Surg. Med.*, **2**, 37-42
12. Apfelberg, D. B., Flores, J. T., Maser, M. R. and Lash, H. (1983). Analysis of complications of argon laser treatment of port wine haemangiomas with reference to striped technique. *Lasers Surg. Med.*, **2**, 357
13. Gilchrest, B. A., Rosen, S. and Noe, J. M. (1982). Chilling port wine stains improves the response to argon laser treatment. *Plast. Reconstr. Surg.*, **69**(2), 278-83
14. Cosman, B. (1982). Role of retreatment in minimal power argon laser therapy for port wine stains. *Lasers Surg. Med.*, **2**, 43-57
15. Greenwald, J., Rosen, S., Anderson, R. R., Harrist, T., MacFarland, F., Noe, J. and Parrish, J. A. (1981). Comparative histological studies of the tunable dye (at 577 nm) laser and argon laser: The specific vascular effects of the dye laser. *J. Invest. Dermatol.*, **77**, 305-10
16. Hulsbergen-Henning, J. P. and van Gemert, M. J. C. (1983). Port wine stain coagulation experiments with a 540 nm continuous wave dye laser. *Lasers Surg. Med.*, **2**, 205
17. Ratz, J. L., Bailin, P. L. and Levine, H. L. (1982). CO_2 laser treatment of port wine stains: A preliminary report. *J. Dermatol. Surg. Oncol.*, **8**, 1039
18. Kaplan, I. and Giler, S. (1984). *CO_2 laser surgery*. (Berlin: Springer-Verlag)
19. Hall, R. R. (1971). Healing of tissues incised by CO_2 laser. *Br. J. Surg.*, **58**, 222
20. Fidler, J. P. (1981). CO_2 laser excision of thermal burns in children. In Atsumi,

K. and Nimsakul, N. (eds). *Laser Tokyo*. Proceedings of 4th Congress of the International Society for Laser Surgery, **24,** 15

21. Bailin, P. L., Ratz. J. L. and Lutz-Nagey, L. (1981). CO_2 laser modification of Mohs' surgery. *J. Dermatol. Surg. Oncol.*, **4,** 243
22. Brunner, R., Landthaler, M., Haina, D., Waidelich, W. and Braun-Falco, O. (1985). Treatment of benign, semi-malignant and malignant skin tumours with the Nd:YAG laser. *Lasers Surg. Med.*, **5**(2), 105–10
23. Levine, H. L. and Bailin, P. L. (1982). Carbon dioxide laser treatment of cutaneous haemangiomas and tattoos. *Arch. Otolaryngol.*, **108,** 236–8
24. Bailin, P. L., Ratz, J. L. and Levine, H. L. (1980). Removal of tattoos by CO_2 laser. *J. Dermatol. Surg. Oncol.*, **6,** 997–1001
25. Mester, E., Mester, A. S. and Mester, A. (1985). Biomedical effects of laser application. *Lasers Surg. Med.*, **5,** 31
26. Surinchak, J. S., Laago, M. L., Bellamy, R. F., Stuck, B. E. and Belkin, M. (1983). Effects of low level energy lasers on the healing of full thickness skin defects. *Lasers Surg. Med.*, **2,** 267
27. Raab, O. (1900). Uber die wirkung fluoreszirenden stoffe und infusoria. *Z. Biol.*, **39,** 524
28. Lipson, R. L., Baldes, E. J. and Olsen, A. M. (1961). Haematoporphyrin derivative: A new aid of endoscopic detection of malignant disease. *J. Thorac. Cardiovasc. Surg.*, **42,** 623
29. Carruth, J. A. S. and McKenzie, A. L. (1985). Preliminary report of a pilot study of photoradiation therapy for the treatment of superficial malignancies of the skin, head and neck. *Eur. J. Surg. Oncol.*, **11,** 47–50

3
CRYOSURGERY

R. P. R. DAWBER

'Today, cryosurgery is a surgical modality essential in the armamentarium of the dermatologist who desires the greatest freedom of choice for many lesions, such as dermatofibroma, sebaceous hyperplasia, actinic keratosis, lentigo, leukoplakia, and superficial basal-cell carcinoma, and a valuable alternate method of therapy for other lesions as diverse as verrucae, acne pits, seborrhoeic keratosis, leishmaniasis, and angiomata. Its current popularity has been established during the past two decades and seems due to three factors: (1) development of inexpensive, simple versatile equipment to utilize readily available cryogens; (2) better understanding of cryobiologic principles and development of accurate methods of predicting and measuring proper depth dose with cryosurgery; and (3) dissemination of knowledge about cryosurgery and establishment of courses and training programs to teach cryosurgery to residents and practicing dermatologists[1].'

So writes Douglas Torre, a leading American proponent and exponent of cryosurgery. The proliferation of literature in the fields of cryobiology, cryotechnology and modern standardized cryosurgery suggests that all is new; but this is certainly not so.

'Modern' cryosurgery emerged more than a century ago with the work of Sir James Arnott using salt/ice mixtures. Despite this, even today in some surgical circles, acceptance of cryosurgery has been slow because of the failure to appreciate the destructive nature of freezing techniques using liquid nitrogen or nitrous oxide. Neither have many purely surgical specialists fully appreciated the importance of the lack of connective tissue distortion produced by freezing. In reviewing the field of cryosurgery it is therefore important to consider its historical and scientific basis.

HISTORICAL BASIS [2,3]

Injury due to cold has been recognized from the earliest times and references to it can be drawn from both civilian and military sources. Historical accounts of the effect of cold climates on various body tissues enable one to reasonably predict the gross changes induced by modern cryosurgical methods. Aryan medicine was concerned with the prevention and cure of illness caused by cold, and Hippocrates noted the effects of cold on the inhabitants of countries with cold climates. In AD 25, Celsus described the appearance of the skin after cold injury and noted that if the injury was severe, dry gangrene supervened. The loss of sensation which accompanies injury was described by Galen (AD 70) in his treatise 'Pain as a means of diagnosis'. Military campaigns in mountainous regions of the ancient world produced cold injuries in endemic proportions. The Carthaginian mercenaries in Hannibal's army which crossed the Alps in 218 BC found that smearing their bodies with oil was an effective means of preventing frost-bite, which nevertheless took a heavy toll. The forces of Alexander the Great found similar protection using sesame juice. Several centuries later a medical diarist, Dr James Thatcher, noted the serious losses of American forces during the War of Independence. He recorded that on one sortie 500 troops were 'slightly frozen' after a night in the open. In the Napoleonic wars, Napoleon's surgeon-general, Von Larrey, made detailed observations of the effects of cold on his patients. He described erythema and blistering of the skin after freezing, and also noted that gangrene was not an inevitable consequence of freezing, if exposure was not prolonged. Uneventful healing of these wounds was also described. Casualties in later campaigns were numerous, amounting to 115 000 in World War One.

Cryosurgery, or the deliberate destruction of diseased tissue by cold in a controlled manner, was first used when suitable refrigerants became available in the nineteenth century. Dr James Arnott, who exhibited his apparatus at the Great Exhibition in 1851, appears to have been the first worker to make use of the therapeutic effects of low temperatures in the destruction of tumours. The use of carbon dioxide snow and liquid air in the treatment of naevi and other skin lesions, at the turn of the century, was followed by the use of other refrigerants – for example, liquid nitrogen. Other therapeutic uses of low temperature in surgery continued to be developed, such as hypothermia, especially in early heart surgery and cryoanaesthesia. Low-temperature saline solutions have been used in the destruction of malignant tumours, and the use of cryosurgery in neurosurgery soon became more widespread, leading to the development of hypophysectomy and the destruction of abnormal basal ganglia. In other fields cryosurgery has been developed in the treatment of a variety of conditions. After the reintroduction of liquid nitrogen this refrigerant was adopted by many dermatologists in the management of neoplastic lesions including basal and squamous cell carcinoma. In gynaecology, cryosurgical techniques have been developed in the treatment of lesions of the cervix and have found a place in ophthalmology for treatment of detached retina and cataract. Cryosurgery is used in otorhinolaryngology, being particularly useful for tonsillectomy in patients with bleeding disorders such as haemophilia and Von Willebrand's disease. This form of treatment has been particularly useful in oral surgery, where the mucous membranes make an ideal moist, smooth surface for freezing; it has been used for leukoplakia, haemangiomas, extravasation cysts, oral neoplasms and many other oral lesions including intractable facial pain where branches of the trigeminal nerve are surgically exposed and frozen.

MECHANISM OF DAMAGE DUE TO COLD INJURY[2]

Cryosurgery can be loosely defined as the deliberate destruction of diseased tissue by freezing in a controlled manner – the controversy regarding whether cryotherapy would be a more representative term can safely be left to the 'semantologists'. Many well-recognized events follow the rapid lowering of temperature in biological systems[2,4].

Factors causing cellular injury

Extracellular ice

When cryosurgery was first introduced it was thought that the main cause of cell death was the formation of ice in the tissues, and the mechanical damage produced as the ice crystals formed. Observation has demonstrated that if cells are frozen *in vitro*, extracellular ice forms first, which gradually squeezes the cells together. It has been difficult to demonstate actual disruption of membranes by this means; however, volume changes in the extra- and intracellular compartments have been measured during freezing and thawing, and the conclusion drawn is that disruption of cell membranes must occur. It appears that extracellular ice formation alone is not sufficient to kill cells: the temperature changes during cryosurgery are so rapid that intracellular ice formation is inevitable as well, this being physically very destructive.

Hypertonic damage

When extracellular ice is formed in association with cell suspension *in vitro*, the amount of extracellular water decreases, causing an increase in concentration of solutes in the remaining fluid. Changing osmotic gradients between cells and extracellular fluids are therefore produced, which lead to passage of electrolytes out of the cells causing a decrease in cell volume and a disruption of cell membranes. It has been shown that when a certain concentration is reached, normally intracellular components – for example, haemoglobin in red blood cells – pass out of the cell causing irreversible damage. Rapid electrolyte transfer has also been incriminated as the cause of damage to cell proteins and enzyme systems, and it is generally accepted that the temperature gradients produced during cryosurgery cause damage by this means, especially during the reverse process of thawing.

Sensitization

In experiments using red blood cells it has been shown that gross cell damage is produced even if hypertonic conditions necessary for disruption are not achieved. It has therefore been postulated that this sensitization damage is the result of disruption of phospholipids in cell membranes, but this has not been confirmed by other workers. It may be that events taking place during thawing, for example reversed osmotic gradients, may give rise to this form of damage.

Intracellular ice

Extracellular ice formation, and sensitization damage, can only occur when freezing is slow, i.e. when differential freezing in different parts of a system is allowed to occur. When very rapid freezing takes place intracellular ice formation occurs, and it is widely believed that this gives rise to cellular death even though cells assume a remarkably normal appearance immediately after thawing. Damage to cell organelles such as mitochondria and endoplasmic reticulum has been postulated to be the cause of injury from intracellular ice. The size of the ice crystals is probably important; the larger the crystals, the greater the damage. Most of the evidence supports the general principle that intracellular ice is lethal. It is probably that recrystallization of ice during the slow thaw after cryosurgery is responsible for tissue destruction, this process being as important as the initial freeze in causing cell death.

Circulatory changes [2,3,5]

Many authorities feel that as important as the initial freeze/thaw events in causing cell and tissue death are: (a) the circulatory (capillary and lymphatic) malfunction associated with the early endothelial damage and oedema; and (b) the capillary and venous occlusion seen several days after treatment, leading to anoxia, further cell death and tissue necrosis.

Immunological events

Cryosurgery has been shown to excite immunological reaction against tumour cells. Lymphocytes and serum from tumour-bearing animals receiving a single cryosurgical dose have demonstrated greater cytotoxicity to an identical tumour in a syngeneic animal than lymphocytes and serum from an untreated animal. This response has been shown to be tissue-specific and stimulated by the release of tumour-specific antigen either during or after freezing. Other workers have observed the effects of an immune reaction after cryosurgery of tissues such as the prostate. Whether such events are important in human cutaneous cryosurgery remains to be proven.

Histological changes

Immediately after freezing, very few cytological abnormalities are evident. Within 30 minutes, cells show pyknotic nuclei, oedema and coarsely granular and often vacuolated cytoplasm. At the edge of the frozen area the cells have eosinophylic cytoplasm with small basophilic nuclei. By 1 hour, dermal vascular damage and oedema appear. Later, changes are those seen in any acutely ischaemic area. The cellular infiltrate consists mainly of polymorphonuclear leukocytes, but also some lymphocytes and plasma cells, mostly at the edge of the treatment ice field. Resolution begins within 3 days.

Routine cryosurgical freeze schedules do not lead to connective tissue distortion[6]. Local nerve damage does consistently occur[7], with myelin and axons appearing to be quite sensitive to cold; however, in view of the resistance of the neural connective tissue sheaths to cold injury, normal regeneration is the rule within a few months, apart from with prolonged or repeat freezes, which may cause permanent nerve damage.

Refrigerants and equipment

Since the nineteenth century, when it became possible to produce and utilize common gases in different phases at various times, several refrigerants have been in vogue. The boiling point of carbon dioxide is $-79\,°C$ and liquid nitrogen $-196\,°C$; nitrous oxide in closed probe systems (Joule-Thomson cooling effect) can cool probe tips to $-70\,°C$. Liquid nitrogen is now the commonest agent used, mainly because it is relatively cheap, widely available, easy to store and quick and easy to use in routine clinical practice; also liquid nitrogen spray and probes give a more rapid rate of freeze (greater cell death) than the other agents. In clinical practice one rarely needs to produce temperatures lower than $-50\,°C$ to produce consistent cell death.

The commonest equipment in use for routine clinical practice is designed to utilize liquid nitrogen as a refrigerant (Figure 3.1).

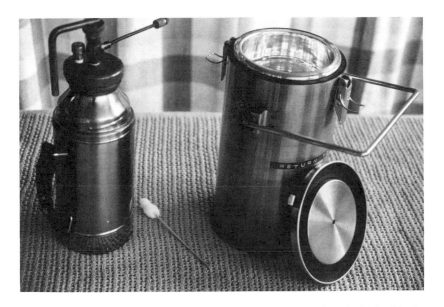

FIGURE 3.1 Commonly used cryosurgery equipment – a handheld liquid nitrogen spray unit (left) with a cotton-wool swab (centre) for the dip technique using a Dewar flask (right) containing liquid nitrogen

'Dip' technique

This long-used method employs either a cotton wool swab or copper discs with insulated handles: the swab or disc is dipped into a robust metal Dewar flask containing liquid nitrogen and then applied to the area to be treated (Figure 3.1). The time of application depends on the size and nature of the lesions to be treated; to maintain relatively long tissue freezing, repeat dipping and reapplication may be necessary. It is very difficult to standardize this technique in view of the many variables – ambient temperature, the pressure applied, distance the dip instrument travels from Dewar flask to the lesion, 'dripping' of liquid nitrogen. This technique is considered to be only suitable for use in benign superficial conditions. 'Artistry' and experience are essential if consistently good cure rates are to be achieved with this method – which has been used successfully by dermatologists for many decades. If premalignant and malignant integumentary lesions are to be treated then modern standardized equipment is required.

For routine outpatient cryosurgery, most dermatologists prefer a small hand-held spray unit (Figure 3.1), or a compact tabletop unit, capable of either spray or cryoprobe application; the former are by far the commonest used in clinical practice. For details of the various commercially produced units available, the reader is referred to more detailed texts[3]. Most units allow for variation in the 'width' of the

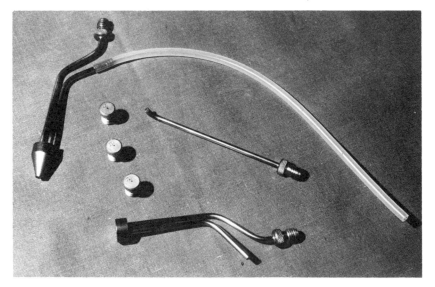

FIGURE 3.2 Various sized 'screw-in' spray and probe attachments for use with the unit shown in Figure 3.1

spray and have probe attachments of different sizes to equate with the size of the area to be treated (Figure 3.2). The probes are generally cylindrical, preferably with flat contact surfaces; they are particularly useful when pressure is needed, for example with vascular lesions and for areas where 'open' spray is a problem (around the eye, the mouth and the vagina); also very small lesions can be treated with pointed probes since spray techniques give too wide an icefield and therefore greater morbidity.

Since liquid nitrogen equipment has largely superseded other instruments utilizing carbon dioxide snow, or nitrous oxide cooling (Joule-Thomson effect) for dermatological lesions, these will not be considered here. The techniques are described in detail elsewhere[3].

Various items of auxiliary equipment are important if the full range of cryosurgical techniques is to be employed:

1. Truncated non-conducting cones[8] are frequently employed to limit surface application of the spray (Figure 3.3a,b). For small lesions, if carefully localized spray is required, auroscope cones can be used. This method gives a very rapid rate of temperature decrease which is probably more destructive than the open spray technique.

2. To protect the orbit of the eye when eyelid tumours are to be treated a plastic eyelid retractor is essential; if one is not available, a plastic spoon without coarse edges may suffice.

3. Monitoring devices[3]. If only benign and relatively flat and small premalignant and malignant lesions are to be treated, then monitoring equipment is unnecessary since no physical instrument can measure adequate cell death. The treatment of deep or large tumours requires careful 'depth dose' monitoring equipment[3] – these are most commonly a pyrometer-thermocouple combination; some methods employ electrical impedance or tissue resistance-measuring devices which in principle have the advantages of measuring actual freezing; only thin, inexpensive electrodes are needed, and many areas of the tumour can be monitored with a single electrode.

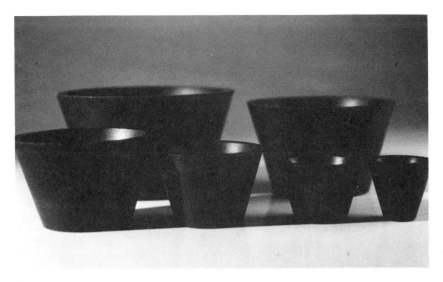

a

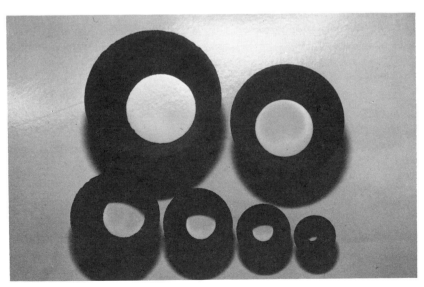

b

FIGURE 3.3 Non-conducting cones used in the conespray technique: (**a**) side view, and (**b**) top view to show the various sizes

CLINICAL EFFECTS

In general, surgical methods of treatment require only simple general explanation to the patient, since most individuals have clear concepts of what to expect in the healing phase after a cut or a heat burn. This is not true for cold injury and therefore each patient needs to be given very careful details of the inflammatory events occurring in the few days after treatment. Because of this, many departments produce a patient leaflet of the type shown in Figure 3.4, which is always used as a vehicle (*never* a substitute) for careful explanation of the skin changes that will be seen.

Pain

The patient usually feels a burning sensation during freezing and thawing. Any pain experienced is usually transient due to the anaesthetizing effect of freezing[7]. Local anaesthesia is not required for short freeze times but may be indicated when treating malignant lesions or for patients thought to have a low pain threshold. Deep treatments on the forehead may occasionally produce migraine-like headaches, and periungual treatment produces relatively greater discomfort than other digital sites.

Inflammation

Some degree of erythema and oedema is to be expected with all cryosurgery treatments and in areas where the skin is lax – periorbital skin, lips, labia majora and penis – oedema may be pronounced. Prolonged freezing schedules may produce blister formation; even short freeze times may cause such changes in atrophic skin.

Because this acute inflammation was thought to be unnecessary to obtain good cure rates, for many years the author has advocated pre- and post-treatment (3–5 days) anti-inflammatory therapy with sol. aspirin 300–600 mg up to four times daily and Dermovate (clobetasol propionate) cream daily to the treated area. The value of this has been confirmed by objective assessment[9].

89

TREATMENT OF SKIN CONDITIONS BY FREEZING

Freezing as a method for treating some skin abnormalities has been in use for more than 150 years. Modern technology has allowed us to get much higher success rates than with older methods; — the machine used to treat your skin is a product of modern technology which carefully controls a very cold liquid, liquid nitrogen, such that it can be sprayed or touched onto any area of skin that needs the treatment. This medical science is called cryosurgery. The particular advantage of the treatment is that it replaces the need for a surgical operation; also under most circumstances it does not leave permanent scars.

In effect, the treatment is a carefully controlled cold burn. The actual procedure may simply cause vague **soreness** or **pain** — this depends on the length of the freeze and the area being treated. After treatment marked redness always occurs together with some swelling; the degree of swelling also depends on the site of treatment and its duration. These changes usually only last for a few days. In some people, particularly where the skin is rather thin and sensitive, a **water (or blood) blister** may form and fluid may discharge. If a blister does form, simply let out the fluid with a sterile pointed instrument; repeat this until the blister no longer refills. If you are prescribed a cream to use, apply it twice daily on any clean dry dressing — unless instructed differently; small areas can be covered with an elastoplast type dressing. If you have not received a prescription, use any antiseptic cream twice daily to avoid the small chance of infection occurring.

Once the fluid discharge or blistering stage is over — usually a few days unless the condition of your skin necessitates prolonged freezing — a crust or scale may form.

If undue discomfort or pain occurs after the treatment then Sol. aspirin tabs 2 three times daily for 3-5 days usually helps; aspirin also helps by limiting the swelling and speeding the healing time.

If any change should occur that has not been explained by the above, or the doctor who treated you, please ring:—

Hospital: . . . .

Tel. No.: . . . .

Extension: . . . .

and explain the problem to the nurse or doctor who answers.

FIGURE 3.4 Patient information leaflet used to explain the skin changes that occur during treatment

CLINICAL USES

During the past 20 years the number of conditions found to be sensitive to cryosurgical treatment has been considerable. Table 3.1 shows a list of lesions treatable by cryosurgery[1,3,5].

In an attempt to standardize the treatment used for different lesions at varying sites, and so that we can further our knowledge of the relative sensitivity or resistance of differing lesions to cryosurgery, we have adopted a 'spot' freeze technique; this enables medical personnel of varying degrees of experience to obtain the same results.

The spot freeze technique involves first defining the size of the field to be treated (as with radiotherapy) and then inducing ice formation within that field by liquid nitrogen spray – large lesions are divided into overlapping circles of 2 cm diameter using a skin marker. The liquid nitrogen spray (e.g. 'C' spray of CryAC Units, Brymill Corp.) is held approximately 1 cm from the skin surface in the centre of a 2 cm circle and spraying commences; the white 'iceline' is allowed to extend outwards until it fills the circle – this icefield is then 'held' for a measured time by continuing the spray with a sufficient jet pressure to maintain the iceline. The measured time will depend entirely on the nature of the lesion; once the time is completed, spraying is stopped and thawing commences. Each 2 cm circle is treated similarly.

A single freeze and thaw is termed a freeze–thaw cycle (FTC); malignant lesions usually receive two, sometimes three, FTCs, the intervening thaw time being at least three times the duration of the initial freeze. Evidently treatment fields of less than 2 cm diameter do not require to be divided up.

The time added after icefield formation must be learned by experience, but will vary with the size, site and type of pathology. The record in the hospital notes is usually made, for example, as follows:

LN_2 : Single icefield : 1 × 15 s
(Liquid nitrogen : Single < 2 cm : 1 FTC × Time after ice
formed)

This schedule is typical of that used for a small flat plaque of Bowen's disease of the skin. Viral warts may require as little as

TABLE 3.1   Lesions treated by cryosurgery (modified from Torre[1])

Cryosurgery treatment of choice

Basal cell carcinoma	Mucocele
(superficial multicentric type)	Porokeratosis (actinic)
Keratosis (actinic)	Porokeratosis (plantar)
Lentigo (actinic, benign)	Sebaceous hyperplasia
Leukoplakia	Verruca (digitate)

Cryosurgery an alternative method of treatment (sometimes combined with other methods)

Acne pits	Keratosis (arsenic)
Acne pustules and cysts	Keratosis (thick seborrhoeic)
Acrochordon	Leiomyoma
Adenoma sebaceum (Pringle)	Leishmaniasis
Angiomas	Lentigo maligna
Angiofibroma	Lentigo maligna melanoma
Angiokeratoma	Lupus erythematosus
Basal cell carcinoma[11] (Figure 3.5)	Lupus vulgaris
Bowen's disease	Mastocytoma
Carbuncle	Molluscum contagiosum
Chloasma	Neurofibroma
Chondrodermatitis	Naevoid basal cell epitheliomata
Clear cell acanthoma	(Gorlin)
Condylomata acuminata	Naevus (epithelial)
Cylindroma	Porokeratosis (Mibelli)
Digital myxoid cyst[14] (Figure 3.6)	Prurigo nodularis
Eccrine poroma	Pseudo-pyogenic granuloma
Elastosis perforans serpiginosa	Pyogenic granuloma
Eosinophilic granuloma	Rhinophyma
Erythroplasia of Queyrat	Sarcoid
Granuloma annulare	Squamous cell carcinoma
Granuloma (mycobacterial)	Steatocystoma multiplex
Hidradenoma	Syringoma
Hidradenitis	Tattoos[12]
Histiocytoma	Trichoepithelioma
Ingrowing toenail	Verruca plana
Intraepidermal of Jadassohn	Verruca plantaris
Keloid[13]	Verruca vulgaris
Keratoacanthoma	Xanthelasma

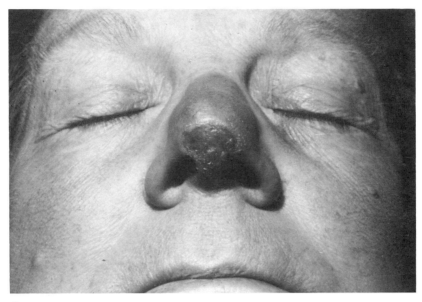

a

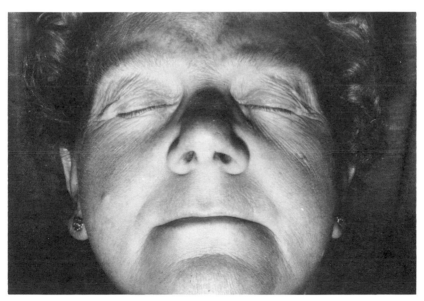

b

FIGURE 3.5 Basal cell carcinoma of the tip of the nose (**a**) before treatment, scab removed, and (**b**) 3 months later

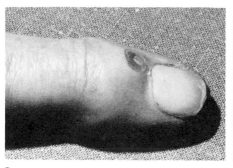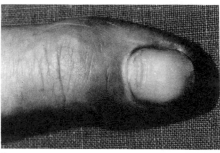

a   b

FIGURE 3.6   Ruptured digital myxoid cyst (**a**) before and (**b**) 6 weeks after treatment

4–5 s, whilst malignant lesions need up to 30 s. Times of less than 30 s do not cause connective tissue distortion and scarring[10].

We have tested the adequacy of the spot freeze method in experiments on the flank skin of pigs[10] and shown consistent cell killing and satisfactory temperature levels within the field of treatment (Figure 3.7). The method is exactly repeatable from patient to patient and site to site; if, following a particular schedule, the treated lesion is not cured, the time of treatment can be lengthened – also whichever doctor sees the case at follow-up, the exact treatment procedure is known and can be specifically modified.

Many other techniques are available involving varying spray methods for treating large lesions and liquid nitrogen probe methods[3]. The important factor is to gain experience with whatever techniques are to be learned by (a) experimenting on skin of cheap meats or other animal tissue, e.g. pigs' feet, available from most meat retailers; (b) working with an animal 'model' where possible; (c) observing experienced operators in practice. This is particularly important if malignant lesions are to be treated since much of the therapeutic failure with small basal and squamous epitheliomata can be ascribed to poor technique.

As with all surgical treatments, accurate diagnosis is essential before cryosurgery is used; this evidently does not mean biopsy of all lesions prior to freezing, since clinical diagnosis will often be adequate, particularly with benign lesions and many basal cell car-

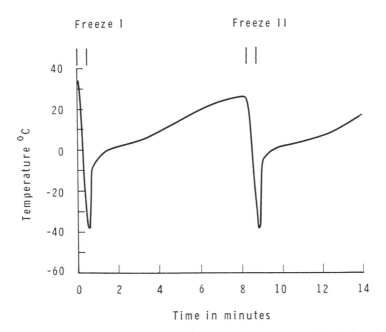

FIGURE 3.7 Temperature changes measured (thermocouple) during $2 \times 20\,s$ freeze–thaw cycles (pig flank; liquid nitrogen spray)

cinomas. As with radiotherapy, wrong diagnosis may lead to 'blurring' of physical signs, for example with melanotic lesions, and may facilitate tumour spread before the diagnosis becomes obvious.

SOME ADVANTAGES AND DISADVANTAGES

Obviously many of the conditions listed in Table 3.1 as being curable by cryosurgery are amenable to other surgical methods; the modality chosen will often depend on the skills available in the department to which the patient has been referred.

Cryosurgery has the advantage over all other modes of being quick, cheap and easy to learn and to carry out; usually sterile surgical facilities are not required and treatment can be initiated even in the presence of bacterial infection, e.g. ingrowing toenail. The fact that post-treatment connective tissue distortion does not generally occur makes cryosurgery advantageous where scarring would be progressively troublesome e.g. perianal, penile, vulval, and periorbital skin; also over joints where a full range of movement can be expected to be retained even after treatment of malignancy with two or three FTCs.

Cartilage necrosis is extremely rare after freezing; therefore ear, eyelid and nasal lesions give good cosmetic results after cryosurgery[15]. It should be remembered that the only consistent exemption to this dogma is cartilage already invaded by tumour – even if good cure is obtained, a cartilage defect may occur.

Anything but the shortest freeze schedules will give pigment changes in the treated area – hyperpigmentation with very short freezes and at the edge of more aggressively treated areas; hypopigmentation occurs after prolonged freezing, e.g. >5s after icefield formation, and may be permanent; therefore cryosurgery is less valuable in patients with racially dark skin – e.g. Asian or Negroid; and 'exposed part' lesions in Caucasian whites who tan darkly on sun exposure.

Temporary impairment of sensation in the treatment area is common after freezing[3]; only rarely will the patient be aware of this. Such nerve ending damage can be expected to disappear within a few months, apart from after 'malignancy regimes' using two or three FTCs. At sites such as the finger pulp and lip margin permanent sensory loss may give important functional impairment, but in other sites it is generally of no significance. Though nerve trunk damage and 'distant' sensory and motor loss have been recorded they are very rare and reversible, usually within a few months.

A rare side-effect of cryosurgery is delayed bleeding; this may be due to granulation tissue formation as in pyogenic granuloma, or from erosion of a small artery. The former may require no more than pressure to abort it, or chemical treatment (e.g. silver nitrate) or electrocautery. A patent bleeding artery requires tying off with an appropriate suture.

References

1. Torre, D. (1985). Cutaneous cryosurgery: current state of the art. *J. Dermatol. Surg. Oncol.*, **11**, 292–5

2. Shepherd, J. P. and Dawber, R. P. R. (1982). Cryosurgery: history and scientific basis. *Clin. Exp. Dermatol.*, **7**, 321–8
3. Zacarian, S. A. (1985). *Cryosurgery for Skin Cancer and Cutaneous Disorders*. (St Louis: C. V. Mosby)
4. Breitbart, E. W. (1983) Cryosurgery: method and results. *Hautarzt*, **34**, 612–19
5. Dawber, R. P. R. (1979). Cryotherapy. In Rook, A., Wilkinson, D. S. and Ebling, F. J. G. (Eds). *Textbook of Dermatology*, 3rd Edn. (Oxford: Blackwell), pp. 2344–6
6. Shepherd, J. P. and Dawber, R. P. R. (1984). Wound healing and scarring after cryosurgery. *Cryobiology*, **21**, 157–69
7. Sonnex, T. S., Jones, R. L., Weddell, A. G. and Dawber, R. P. R. (1985). Long term effects of cryosurgery on cutaneous sensation. *Br. Med. J.*, **290**, 188–90
8. Torre, D. (1978). Cryosurgical treatment of epitheliomas using the cone-spray technique. *J. Dermatol. Surg. Oncol.*, **4**, 561–4
9. Hindson, T. C., Spiro, J. and Scott, L. V. (1985). Clobetasol proprionate ointment reduces inflammation after cryotherapy. *Br. J. Dermatol.*, **112**, 599–602
10. Shepherd, J. P. and Dawber, R. P. R. (1984). Wound healing and scarring after cryosurgery. *Cryobiology*, **21**, 157–69
11. Zacarian, S. A. (1983). Cryosurgery of cutaneous carcinoma. *J. Am. Acad. Dermatol.*, **9**, 947–66
12. Colver, G. B. and Dawber, R. P. R. (1984). Tattoo removal using liquid nitrogen cryospray. *Clin. Exp. Dermatol.*, **9**, 364–6
13. Shepherd, J. P. and Dawber, R. P. R. (1982). The response of hypertrophic and keloid scars to cryosurgery. *Plast. Reconstr. Surg.*, **70**, 677–82
14. Dawber, R. P. R., Sonnex, T., Leonard, J. and Ralfs, I. (1982). Myxoid cysts of the finger; treatment by liquid nitrogen cryosurgery. *Clin. Exp. Dermatol.*, **8**, 153–7
15. Burge, S. M., Shepherd, J. P. and Dawber, R. P. R. (1984). Effect of freezing the helix and the rim or edge of the human and pig ear. *J. Dermatol. Surg. Oncol.*, **10**, 816–19

4
COSMETIC SURGERY

E. HANEKE

INTRODUCTION

There is a growing demand for high-level skin surgery. However, the subject of cosmetic surgery performed by dermatologists is a matter of controversy between dermatologists, general surgeons, maxillofacial surgeons, and plastic surgeons, at least in some countries. Due to his profound knowledge of the skin's biology and pathology the dermatologist is not only able to perform simple surgical operations but also to consider completely different treatment modalities including surgical approaches[1,2].

REMOVAL OF COSMETICALLY EMBARRASSING LESIONS

Pigmented lesions

Lentigo simplex

Simple lentigines are small, round, dark brown to black spots. Removal of the pigment-containing epidermis is sufficient. The lesion is gently heated to burn the epidermis which then is wiped away with a cotton gauze. Treatment is by hot cautery or light electrodesiccation. Alternative treatment modalities are shave excision, cryotherapy, laser, chemical cautery, and dermabrasion.

Naevocellular naevi (NCN)

Treatment of acquired naevi is by surgical excision. The scar can often be placed into a skin fold and within months will become inconspicuous. Shave excision is widely used in some countries and often gives excellent cosmetic results if no repigmentation occurs.

Congenital NCN are usually much larger and darker. They have a risk of malignant degeneration, particularly giant naevi. Small congenital NCN are excised; if they cannot be removed by a one-step operation serial excisions can be performed (Figures 4.1 and 4.2). Fusiform excisions are taken from the centre so that the scar from the previous operation is always in the middle of the next excision. It is essential to avoid wound dehiscence and scar widening. Two-layered sutures are therefore necessary. PDS, vicryl or Dexon hold strong for some weeks and are used as running dermal sutures. 'Subcutaneous' (fat) sutures are of no value except to coapt deep wound spaces. Either single through-and-through or running sutures are used for final closure. Monofil threads can be left in place for 2 weeks or even longer if put in the remaining NCN. Adhesive strips will further facilitate wound healing and coaptation. A period of 4–8 months has to elapse between the excisions[3].

Either serial excisions or multi-step procedures including free grafts are recommended to treat giant naevi and to avoid melanoma development. Cosmetically highly acceptable results have been

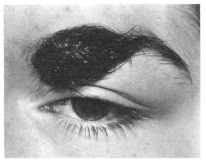 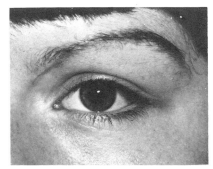

a **b**

FIGURE 4.1 Deeply pigmented hairy congenital naevus in a 17-year-old girl: (**a**) before operation; (**b**) after excision and closure with a 6/0 prolene running intracutaneous suture

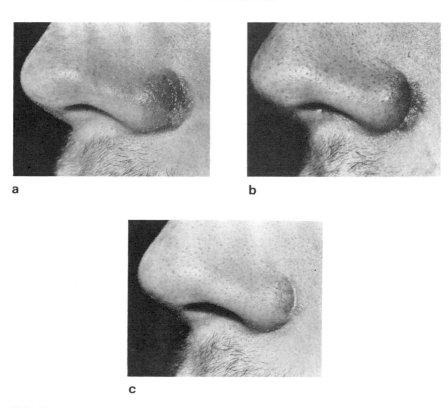

a   b

c

FIGURE 4.2   Congenital naevus in a 15-year-old boy: (**a**) before operation; (**b**) after first excision along the crease of the ala nasi; (**c**) after two full-thickness excisions and shave excision of the remaining fourth of the naevus

achieved by high-speed dermabrasion provided it is performed during the first 6–8 weeks of life. Removal of the superficial cells leads to a nearly complete disappearance of pigmentation; the skin shows an inconspicuous superficial scar (Figure 4.3). Repigmentation, if at all, is light and spotty. The deeply pigmented lesions of neurocutaneous melanosis cannot be treated successfully with dermabrasion.

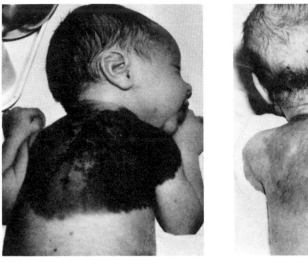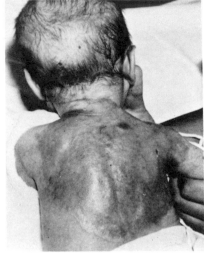

a   b

FIGURE 4.3   Giant congenital naevus of a 9-day-old boy: (**a**) before operation; (**b**) 14 days after high-speed dermabrasion of the entire naevus at the age of 11 days

Senile lentigines

The treatment of choice in case of diagnostic uncertainty is complete removal by shave excision. It is wise to use a certain amount of local anaesthetic to elevate the lesion to be removed. Trichloroacetic acid, 35% or 50%, gives a mild peel usually sufficient to eliminate this pigmentation.

Café au lait spots

A chemical peel may also be tried for café au lait spots of neurofibromatosis, though it is difficult to obtain cosmetically satisfactory permanent results; dermabrasion is not consistently successful.

Chloasma

Chloasma is due to pigmentary incontinence; therefore chemical peels largely fail to give satisfactory results. Instead the inflammation associated with healing after the peel may even worsen the condition by adding postinflammatory hyperpigmentation to the original chloasma. If at all, weak peeling agents such as 25% trichloracetic acid may be used several times at monthly intervals, starting in autumn; using potent sun-screens and avoiding both direct sun irradiation and sharp cold wind are recommended.

Vascular lesions

Spider naevi

Electrocoagulation of the central vessel will usually cure the small lesion. A thin electrical needle is lightly held on the centre and only then does the nurse slowly turn on the high-frequency current. The vessel is coagulated when the needle has sunk in.

Telangiectasia

Telangiectases of large diameter are best sclerosed using 0.5–1% ethoxysclerol (polidocanol) and a 20- or 30-gauge injection needle. Electrocoagulation is best for smaller vessels. The results are generally better the lower the current.

Sunburst vessels

The treatment of choice of these venous blemishes of the legs is sclerotherapy. Ethoxysclerol 0.5–1% is commonly used in Europe, and 23.4% sodium chloride solution is more often used in the USA.

A 1 ml tuberculin syringe with a 30-gauge needle is used. The needle is placed in an acute angle on the skin with the bevel of the needle facing downward and its tip 3–4 mm from the vessel to be injected. The needle is gently moved forward. Light pressure to the piston of the syringe will produce blanching of the vessel as soon as it is cannulated. When 0.1–0.5 ml is injected one can see that a large portion of the arborizing vessel blanches. The sclerosing solution is to damage vessel walls and to lead to permanent occlusion. Despite much experience it is not always possible to cannulate tiny vessels. A minute amount of ethoxysclerol, about 0.05 ml of a 0.25–0.5% solution, may then be placed into their close surroundings. No necrosis will develop if both the concentration and amount are very low. A cellulose roll or cotton ball is applied to the injected vessels with pressure and fixed with adhesive tape to prevent blood from filling the vessel and leaking into the dermal connective tissue. A compression dressing is applied for 24–48 hours. Ordinary elastic bandages are used for the lower leg while foam-rubber bandages have to be used for the thigh since elastic bandages usually do not remain in place.

Cherry angioma

Laser, electrocoagulation, chemical cautery and cryotherapy achieve comparable results.

Epithelial lesions

Milia

Treatment of choice is to remove the roof of each milium and express the content with its epithelial lining. Unroofing is simplest with a No. 11 scalpel blade, an electrical needle or a 12-gauge injection needle. If carefully done no scarring will occur.

Skin tags

The simplest treatment is grasping skin tags with fine forceps and cutting them at their base with scissors. Electrodesiccation and chemical cautery are alternative methods.

Sebaceous hyperplasia

A fusiform excision closed with a running intracutaneous suture gives the best cosmetic result. Chemical cautery with liquefied phenol (88-90%) may be tried, but since the lesion usually reaches down to the deep reticular dermis this procedure has often to be repeated and the scar may be hypopigmented.

Seborrhoeic keratosis (basal cell papilloma)

Shave excision under local anaesthesia is the treatment of choice. A No. 10 scalpel blade is held against the border of the seborrhoeic keratosis. The skin is stretched with the thumb and index finger and the lesion cut at its base with sweeping strokes of the scalpel. This leaves a completely even superficial wound. Haemostasis is obtained with 20% aqeous solution of aluminium chloride. Scarring is absent or minimal.

Curettage with a spoon-shaped or ring curette is most commonly described as the easiest treatment. This leaves a raw wound surface, and considerable tearing forces are exerted to the skin during curettage. Elastotically degenerated skin may break and suffusion may occur leaving considerable pigmentation that only very slowly fades.

Viral warts

Surgical treatment generally is not an adequate approach. However, filiform warts on the face, lips and eyelids may be very ugly. Shave excision and slight electrodesiccation safely cure these lesions. No permanent scarring should occur.

Syringomas

If there are only a few syringomas, fusiform excision respecting the relaxed skin tension lines (RSTL) and skin closure with 7/O monofil sutures give excellent results.

Cysts

For epidermoid cysts, local anaesthesia is obtained by injecting the anaesthetic around the cyst. A linear incision or a narrow fusiform skin excision are planned. The incision must not be carried down to the subcutis since the cyst is usually located within the dermis. Careful dissection of the epithelial and fibrous sac without severing it can be very difficult, but should always be tried in order to completely remove the cyst and avoid wound infection.

Wound closure is by a two-layered suture. Occasionally a subcutaneous suture is necessary to avoid a deep wound space that would fill with blood and carry the risk of infection.

Acutely inflamed cysts are first incised, drained and treated with an antibiotic active against staphylococci; 4–6 weeks after complete healing should elapse before cyst removal.

Tricholemmal cysts have more resistant walls; their removal is therefore much simpler. After a small skin incision the dermis is spread with blunt scissors until the smooth whitish cyst wall is seen. The scissor branches are closed and gently forced around the cyst to free it from the surrounding connective tissue. It is then levered up and extruded. The wound is closed with monofil threads.

Dermal and subcutaneous lesions

Xanthelasma

Excision, laser treatment and superficial electrodesiccation have yielded comparable results. Under local anaesthesia the lesion is excised with a fusiform excision and the defect is closed with 7/O monofil sutures. These are removed after 4–5 days. Steristrips are used for another 3–5 days to prevent wound dehiscence. Electrodesiccation is performed very lightly since it is sufficient to remove the overlying epidermis and tips of the papillae. Deep electrocoagulation will result in scars tending to shrink and to remain hypopigmented. Chemical cautery with 50% trichloroacetic acid is also effective.

Adenoma sebaceum (angiofibroma)

Dermabrasion will plane the skin, and re-epithelialization rapidly occurs. Though this method gives the best cosmetic results they are the least permanent. However, dermabrasion may be repeated giving the same good result.

Electrosurgical planing is more radical, but healing takes much longer, hypertrophic scarring may occur, and there is a tendency to recurrence. Recently laser coagulation has given good results.

Neurofibromatosis

When excising raised and pedunculated tumours it has to be appreciated that neurofibromas are soft tumours penetrating the entire dermis and destroying its continuity. Sutures must pass through adequate amounts of normal dermis, but nevertheless wound dehiscence may be a problem. Large overhanging tumours may demand major plastic surgery.

Lipoma

Under local anaesthesia a comparatively small incision is made over the lipoma and the tumour is dissected free from the surrounding normal fat tissue with blunt scissors. Even relatively large lipomas can then be expressed through the small incision. Giant lipomas can be treated with liposuction.

HYPERTRICHOSIS

Bleaching and shaving usually do not give satisfactory results. Cold wax is available for leg hairs. Cosmeticians use hot wax to epilate large hairy areas. Plucking is the best treatment for pseudofolliculitis due to pili recurvati often seen in the beard region of men with curly hair.

Permanent epilation is obtained with a high-frequency machine at the lowest power. Epilating needles are as fine as possible or only the tip is conductive while the sides are insulated (Kromayer needles). This reduces scarring to a minimum. Epilation is not easy and is usually done by a cosmetician. Using a magnifying lens, the epilating needle is inserted into the follicle and gently pushed down until the skin gives some resistance. The current is applied by using a foot pedal. If the hair papilla is destroyed the hair shaft can be easily taken out with a small forceps. After epilation erythematous red papules may occur, resolving within 15 days. The success rate is between 50 and 75%. Many sessions are needed to epilate an area completely. Electrolysis with an electrical forceps is much easier to perform; however, its regrowth rate is much higher and, despite many claims by manufacturers of electrolysis devices, convincing results have not been obtained by most users.

RHINOPHYMA

The operation may be done under general or local anaesthesia, the latter being a combination of infiltration and regional nerve block accomplished with intranasal epimucosal anaesthesia. A bipolar high-frequency machine is used. With a fine noose slowly passed through the hyperplastic tissue from the root to the tip of the nose, 2 mm thick strips of the redundant tissue are removed. The current has to be high enough to cut but the lower the intensity the less bleeding is experienced. Having reached the rough pre-rhinophyma contour of the nose great care is taken not to go too deep, since this will lead to unsightly scarring, hypertrophic scars, or necrosis of the nasal cartilage. The alae nasi are moulded by moving the electrical noose according to the natural impression from the central cheek to the dorsum nasi. During operation the level of tissue removal can be controlled by holding the branches of a forceps on the nose and gently squeezing the skin in between. As long as keratinous debris can be expressed there is no danger of irreversible damage to structures that must not be destroyed. It is better to face the risk of a recurrence than to get scarring.

To avoid possible scarring from electrical burn, removal of the redundant tissue with a scalpel or a razor was proposed[4]. The tissue is removed in small strips and slices. Bleeding is extensive because of the high vascularity. Haemostasis of pulsating vessels is obtained with a bipolar electrical forceps, and human fibrinogen concentrate may stop the profuse bleeding at the end of the operation, providing also a natural dressing and accelerating wound healing[5].

CHELOIDS AND ACNE SCARS

The differentiation between hypertrophic scars, cheloidal scarring and cheloids is somewhat artificial. The risk of recurrence in 'true cheloids' is much higher than in hypertrophic scars[6].

The recurrence risk of at least 50% has to be discussed with the patient. Possible additional treatment modalities such as X-irradiation, intralesional injections of steroid or superoxide dismutase (a metallo-enzyme) have to be assessed. A recurring cheloid will be larger than the original one!

Even the slightest injury must be avoided. Field anaesthesia is obtained by inserting the needle only into the skin that will be excised, together with the cheloid. The anaesthetic is injected into the subcutaneous tissue under the prospective wound margins. The dermis has to be cut with a single stroke. The dermal wound margins must not be touched with any instrument, not even with the finest hooks. These are inserted into the subcutis during mobilization. Wound closure must be achieved without any tension since tension will inevitably result in a recurrence. No flaps are allowed for closure of skin defects from the excision of cheloids. Skin closure is obtained by a running suture at the junction between dermis and subcutis. The suture is removed, about 10 days after operation, since foreign bodies – even absorbable material – stimulate the fibroblastic response. Atraumatic stainless-steel wire sutures are tolerated best. The free ends of the monofil threads are fixed with adhesive tape. Steristrips or butterfly sutures are used for definite coaptation of the dermis and epidermis.

If wound closure cannot be accomplished without tension a free graft is taken. This has to be as thin as possible (Thiersch graft including only epidermis and papillary dermis) to avoid cheloidal scarring of the donor site. The graft is spread over the defect with wide overlapping. It is sutured laterally to the base of the defect (subcutaneous tissue!) and steri-strips are used for fixation of the overlapping portion to the surrounding skin. A light pressure dressing and strict immobilization of the treated area are necessary. If Roentgen therapy is considered the first dose is applied immediately postoperatively by an experienced radiotherapist. Steroid injections are given round the incision line 1 week after operation. Superoxide dismutase is infiltrated around the wound under local anaesthesia in a dosage of 4–8 mg every 2–4 weeks.

Acne scarring usually poses considerable difficulties. Excision is adequate for hypertrophic scars, bridged scars, old fistulae and fibrotic indented scars adherent to the underlying tissue. A No. 11 pointed blade is best suited for small excisions. A two-layered 6/O running intracutaneous PDS suture gives the best result. Steri-strips splint the wound margins together. Round to oval depressed scars up to 3 mm in diameter are punched out. Healing by secondary intention results in a smaller, less depressed scar.

Punch elevation is worthwhile for round to oval scars with a sharp margin and even but depressed bases of normally pigmented skin. A punch 0.5 mm larger than the scar is run through the entire dermis. The cylinder is elevated usually without freeing it from its subcutaneous pedicle and held in place by a 7/O suture, steri-strip or pressure.

The punch replacement technique works best in patients with a few but conspicuous small scars. The scar is removed by a punch, and a full-thickness skin punch including subcutaneous fat is taken from the posterior aspect of the pinna or postauricular skin with a punch that is 0.5 mm larger. This is gently pressed into the primary defect. It has usually to be rotated to find the optimal position to blend in with the surrounding skin. Steri-strips hold the punches in place for a week to 10 days. Since accidental pulling out of the punches may occur some authors use a 7/O suture.

Dermabrasion is used for a large number of small elevated scars. The results in depressed scars are not satisfactory since the normal skin has to be abraded down to the level of the depressions. Therefore, punch elevation is used to elevate deeply impressed scars followed by dermabrasion some 2–6 weeks later to plane the resulting scars. Soft acne scars with smooth margins are effectively treated with injectable collagen.

REMOVAL OF TATTOOS

Accidental tattoos are due to gunpowder, soil, dirt or rubber particles. Immediate treatment within the first 48 hours after the accident will usually remove most of the foreign particles. Under general anaesthesia the whole area is disinfected and brushed with a sterile hand- or tooth-brush until the foreign particles are removed. The bristles of the brush intrude into the wound canal and toss out the foreign particles. During the procedure the skin is rinsed with mercury oxycyanate solution 1:3000.

Particles remaining in the dermis are extruded with the tip of a No. 12 cannula. The brushed skin is gently cleaned with wet cotton pads, covered with antibiotic-impregnated tulle gras and wet compresses which are kept moist during the next 48 hours. Epithelialization readily takes place and is usually complete after 5-8 days[7].

Amateur tattoos usually have the pigment introduced very deeply and irregularly, whereas professional decorative tattoos are more superficial with a clearer appearance. If possible a complete excision is done[2]. Serial excisions are useful for larger tattoos[3].

Where surgical excision is not possible the entire pigment-bearing skin layers have to be removed. Tattoo shops and lay persons use cauterizing agents such as acids, potassium permanganate crystals or even a hot iron.

Salabrasion is simple and cheap, and gives acceptable results in experienced hands. Under local anaesthesia the epidermis is abraded with sandpaper. Cotton gauze is wrapped around a hand-brush, moistened with water and dipped into crystalline table salt. The tattooed skin is stretched and the salt is vigorously rubbed into the dermis until the entire tattoo is dark red. The wound is rinsed, painted with an antimicrobial solution and covered with a light dry dressing. A crust consisting of dried exudate and necrotic dermal tissue with the foreign pigment forms, that is slowly shed leaving a superficial scar. The technique may be capricious since it is difficult to assess the depth of the dye to be removed and the level of tissue injury reached with the hypertonic salt solution.

Dermabrasion allows systematic removal of tissue containing pigment. Light dermabrasion of non-tattooed skin in between hides the outline of the original tattoo. It is easy to see the border of the subcutis and to avoid too deep a defect. Amateur tattoos, being very deep, have sometimes to be dermabraded twice or remaining spots are excised and the dermis is sutured with 5/O vicryl. It is crucial not to create an area of deep wound, in order to avoid hypertrophic scarring, as in a burn scar.

Superficial tattoos have been treated by superficial dermabrasion. Dye particles remaining in the dermis are taken up by macrophages migrating into the dressing. This is changed every day, which is a very painful procedure. The results are excellent when this technique works.

A combination of split-thickness grafts and dermabrasion gives good results in amateur tattoos where the pigment is very deep, but it is very time-consuming[8]. A thin split skin graft is taken over the tattoo and left pedicled. The dermis containing the pigment is dermabraded. The skin graft, if completely free from dye particles, is used to cover the dermabrasion wound and is sutured to the defect. Remaining foreign particles in the split skin are removed by gentle dermabrasion of its undersurface, or excised and the graft sutured in pieces. Healing time is considerably shorter and no hypertrophic scars will develop. Numerous milia and small inclusion cysts often develop but disappear spontaneously or after draining with the tip of a No. 12 injection cannula.

DERMABRASION

Mechanical dermabrasion with rotating machines is now over 80 years old. Speeds up to 60 000 rpm are obtained with the Schreuss Derma III high-speed dermabrader. At this speed the skin behaves like a nearly non-elastic tissue. Dermabrasion tips are serrated steel, diamond fraises, wire or nylon brushes. Practice is necessary for all dermabrasion machines, and the higher the speed the steadier the surgeon's hands and the patient have to be. General anaesthesia is recommended for facial dermabrasion. Serrated steel and coarse diamond fraises are preferentially used for removal of greater amounts of tissue. Broad tips avoid gouging.

The assistant holds the skin taut during dermabrasion. He should wear cotton gloves over rubber gloves for a firmer hold of the skin[9]. The fraise is lightly held against the skin and moved in the long axis of the treatment into the direction of the hand-piece with the operator's thumb resting on the skin. Particular attention has to be paid to eyelids and lips in order to avoid serious lacerations. No hair and no cotton gauze must be within reach of the rotating fraise. Chin and lips are particularly problematic areas. A dental plastic hardening within 5 minutes (Optosil) is moulded over the teeth, gingiva and into the vestibulum, giving firm support to the assistant's hands tautening the lip skin. The eyes are protected with petroleum jelly and a teaspoon. Operator, assistant and nurse have to wear safety shields[9].

The skin is abraded layer by layer but defects reaching down to the reticular dermis will give considerable scarring. Excessive bleeding during dermabrasion is sometimes a particular problem.

For acne, several consecutive dermabrasions may be necessary. Low-speed dermabraders require freezing. The dermabrasion is usually carried out to the end of natural folds or over an entire cosmetic unit of the face.

Postoperative care is important to avoid worsening of the treatment results. Human fibrinogen provides a natural dressing, inhibits oozing and stimulates rapid healing. Antibiotic tulle gras and compresses moistened with physiologic saline avoid sticking of the dressing, drain the exudate and inhibit crust formation. Vigilon, a colloidal polyethylene oxide (4%) suspension which is non-adherent, permeable to air and absorbs moisture, was found to be superior to other occlusive dressings. It permits both a moist environment and absorption of wound exudate.

Biobrane (a synthetic dressing material) sticks to the wound surface and need not be changed. It loosens with wound epithelialization and falls off spontaneously. Superficial dermabrasions re-epithelialize within 5-10 days whereas those for tattoo removal take 4-5 weeks.

Chief indications for dermabrasions are tattoos, acne scars, verrucous epidermal naevi, solar elastosis, and some pigmentations, but also Pringle's adenoma sebaceum, epithelioma adenoides cysticum, rhinophyma, seborrhoeic keratoses, dyskeratosis follicularis Darier, syringoma and many other cosmetic problems[10].

Complications most commonly encountered are pigmentary disturbances, hypertrophic scars, persistent erythema and gouging of skin.

Contraindications are pyoderma and acne pustules. Recurrent herpes simplex may be triggered and give rise to a severe infection comparable to eczema herpeticum. Plane warts must not be treated since inoculation with widespread dissemination will result. Chronic radiodermatitis and burn scars show delayed healing or fail to heal.

CHEMICAL PEEL

Theoretically any cauterant would work, but phenol and trichloroacetic acid are now used preferentially. Major indications are sun-damage, fine wrinkles, and pigmentary disturbances. Persons with fair complexion, solar elastosis and fine to moderate wrinkling are ideal candidates. Dark-skinned people have a tendency to blotchiness after chemical peel.

Phenol peel

Baker's phenol mixture (3 ml liquefied phenol 88-90%, 2 ml tap water, 9 drops liquid soap (lysol, septisol), 3 drops croton oil or camphor) is prepared freshly and stirred before use. The skin is thoroughly defatted with a solvent or soap, ensuring an even penetration of the phenol.

Cotton-tipped applicators, commonly used as a pair, are dipped into the solution. Excess phenol is pressed out and the phenol is evenly painted on the skin. A frost-white colour develops within a few seconds and the application is repeated until the entire area has an even frost. It is convenient to start with the forehead, going on to the cheeks and chin. The peel is done along the ears, below the mandible and beyond the vermillion border to hide the demarcation of peeled and non-peeled skin. A safety margin of 1-4 mm is kept at the ciliary margin to avoid scarring and ectropion formation. Only one cosmetic area is treated about every 15 minutes to avoid cardiotoxic phenol blood levels. At the moment of application a slight burning is felt, soon disappearing due to the local anaesthetic action of phenol. A cool moist compress is put on the treated skin until the whole face is covered with adhesive tape, either micropore or water-proof, starting with the forehead and continuing down to the chin and jaw line sparing only eyes, nostrils and mouth. The tape occlusion increases penetration and augments the peeling effect. The tape must not produce wrinkles, to avoid uneven occlusion. Severe pain usually develops after an hour and requires adequate analgesia.

The tape is removed after 24–48 hours but this again is painful. The skin is greyish or bright red, oedematous and oozing. The eyelids are swollen shut and the lips protrude, giving the patient a frightening appearance. The patient should be warned of that prior to the peel. The oozing face soon becomes crusted. We have the patient keep the crusts soft using antibiotic gauze plus antibiotic cream, and cool moist compresses for the next 2–4 days. When changing the dressing the patient may take a shower and gently wash her face. Since phenol itself is an antiseptic, wound infection is not seen provided there is proper postoperative care and prevention of thick crusts. The scabs gradually fall off during washing but the patient is asked not to deliberately remove or pick them, because this will impair re-epithelialization.

When the crusts are off a smooth erythematous skin is seen that is sensitive to any trauma. Emollients are used overnight and sun blockers at day. Make-up can be worn after 2 weeks. Complete healing takes about 6 months. Sunscreens are used during that time to avoid spotty pigmentation which only responds to a second peel.

Trichloroacetic acid (TCA)

TCA is commonly used at concentrations of 25%, 35%, and 50% (TCA 25, 35 or 50 g, add tap water to 100 ml). The application of TCA is the same as for phenol. 25% TCA is used for eyelids. 35% TCA is usually sufficient for mild solar elastosis and light cross-hatch wrinkling; 50% is for moderate to severe sun damage. To enhance its action tape occlusion may be used. The procedure is carried out more quickly than with phenol. The frost is not as white as that after phenol due to the fact that TCA causes a more intense coagulation of proteins. Therefore, oozing is much less, but removal of tape after occlusion is more painful. Healing is more rapid. TCA is also used to peel small areas such as solar melanosis, flat seborrhoeic keratoses or circumscribed plaque-like elastosis[11].

RHYTIDECTOMY

Rhytidectomy is the excision of skin creases and deep wrinkles, some of which are effectively treated with intradermal collagen injections.

The ageing nose increases in size and droops, with the tip tilting downward. A skin excision on the bridge of the nose can considerably improve the appearance of the drooping nose. Whether or not the patient is a candidate for this simple but efficient technique is tested by taking the skin of the nasal bridge between the index finger and thumb and pinching it. If there is sufficient elevation of the dropped nasal tip a curvilinear incision is made across the bridge just above the level of the medial canthus until about 1 cm from the canthus. A 30–45° back-cut in an inferior and medial direction is made from the lateral edge of the incision. The nasal skin is undermined and pulled upward until the nasal tip is elevated at the desired level. Excess skin is trimmed away. A two-layered skin suture is performed. Up to 10 mm of skin may be excised.

Rhytidectomies may also be performed for single loose pendulous folds and asymmetric creases and wrinkles after tumour excision of the other side of the face.

Frontal rhytidectomy may remove creases and redundant skin. Several fusiform excisions are carried out horizontally on the forehead and vertically between the eyebrows.

Lateral eyebrow lift

The lateral portion of the eyebrows often sinks, giving the face a melancholic expression and exaggerating the sagging of the upper lid. A crescentic excision is performed with its inferior cut running at the margin of the eyebrows. Depending upon the degree of lifting desired, the superior incision will mark a half-moon-shaped excision of 8–12 mm in its greatest width. Separate vertical half-intracutaneous mattress sutures with the knots in the eyebrows will give a scar that is hardly visible.

Face-lift

The ideal candidate is a person with marked sagging and heavy relaxation on a good bony frame with a minimum of fat. Innumerable surgical techniques have been described for a face-lift. Some baselines, however, have to be followed to avoid disastrous complications. All standard face-lift techniques depend basically on two principles: undermining of the skin in the subcutaneous fat and external to the superficial fascia and platysma; closure places tension mainly on the skin.

Patient counselling takes a long time to explain all possible complications. Accurate and realistic preoperative photographs are obligatory. A detailed surgical consent form should be signed by the patient[2].

Anticoagulants such as heparin or dicoumerol, platelet aggregation inhibitors such as acetylsalicylic acid (Aspirin) have to be withdrawn, as well as oestrogens and contraceptive pills.

The face and hair have to be washed for a minimum of 2–3 days preoperatively with an antiseptic detergent. The hair is not shaved except for a small band of 1–2 cm in width where the supra- and postauricular incisions are drawn. A conservative face-lift is recommended for dermatologists performing this surgery. It is usually done under general anaesthesia. Eye salve is put into the conjunctival sac and face and hair are disinfected. The hair is tied into strands and sprayed. The margins of the operation field are taped with Op-Site or another comparable material. The incision lines are marked with a waterproof sterile pencil.

The curved incision of 30–33 cm in length begins in the temple region, extends down slightly anterior to or behind the tragus of the ear, underneath the ear lobe and goes up in the retroauricular crease to the posterior surface of the pinna to finally extend backward into the lower margin of the occipital hair. Masterful camouflage of the incision is essential.

The preauricular incision is cautiously deepened until visualizing the thick fascia which, at this position, is the joining of parotid fascia and the SMAS (superficial musculoaponeurotic system). This deep incision is cautiously extended for 10–20 mm and the skin and sub-cutis are forced medially. Undermining is accomplished mostly with blunt scissors dissection. It should not exceed 6 cm, but in most cases 3–4 cm are sufficient. The subcutaneous fat overlying the platysma, sternocleidomastoid muscle and parotid fascia is carefully removed to expose the SMAS. Five to six plication sutures are placed on each side extending from the infra-auricular to the preauricular area using non-absorbable sutures with buried knots. This is the important deep layer of closure giving support to the skin suture by relieving tension on the elevated skin flap. This deep layer suture can be retracted in a direction independent of the skin, which is particularly important for the submental area.

Before closing the skin a sponge is placed beneath the elevated skin and over the plicated SMAS. After the other side has been operated on in the same way the sponge on the first side is removed to allow a second look for any bleeding vessels and to obtain definite haemostasis. The skin flaps are now ready to be pulled upward and posteriorly. The skin flaps are hooked on and retracted to demonstrate the best position. Cuts are made into the flaps in a perpendicular direction to their free margin and key sutures are placed at the anterior junction of the helix and at the point where the retroauricular incision curves down to the postauricular hair line. Excess skin overlapping the original incision is removed. This results in a flap of only 2–3 cm in width or even less in a conservative face-lift. It is essential to avoid preauricular tension whereas moderate tension is allowed in the region of the temple and postauricularly. Skin closure is accomplished in layers with 4/O vicryl and 6/O prolene. Too great a tension in the temporal and occipital regions may cause temporary alopecia, widening of the scar, or even skin slough. If haemostasis is absolute one may consider not to drain and to only apply a pressure dressing. The majority of face-lift operations usually drain up to 25 ml of blood, serum and interstitial fluid from each side within the first postoperative 48 hours. Haemovac drainage is therefore frequently recommended.

Blunt scissors dissection is now becoming replaced by blunt tunnelling and liposuction. Bleeding has been reduced to negligible levels with this technique, and damage to nerves is extremely rare.

Bleeding is also considerably reduced or completely prevented by using concentrated human fibrinogen. No drains are used after topical fibrinogen glueing. Since the fibrin makes the wound surfaces stick together sutures with very fine threads can be used.

Running intracutaneous 5/O sutures are used in the preauricular incision with a few separate 6/O percutaneous stitches. 4/O sutures are used postauricularly. The scalp incisions may be closed with interrupted 4/O sutures or staples. The wounds are painted with an antiseptic. The incisions are covered with non-sticky Adaptic strips (these strips are metallic on one side).

A firm dressing giving support to the submental area and soft padding behind the pinna is applied using an elastic bandage around the scalp-chin-cheeks-scalp-nape-forehead-occiput.

Percutaneous sutures are cautiously removed after 7 days; those in the mastoid pull area after 10-12 days. The stainless steel staples may remain in place up to 2-3 weeks since no inflammatory reaction has been observed.

More or less prominent cable lines in the submental area giving the appearance of a turkey wattle are due to a hypertrophied mid-portion of the platysma. They may cause a major cosmetic problem in the neck area. The platysma originating from the superficial fasciae of the pectoralis major and deltoid muscles is a broad but thin sheet of striated muscle. It inserts in the mandible and facial skin and subcutaneous tissue. A 2-3 cm incision is made in the transverse submental crease and the skin is elevated from the mental fat pad which is removed so that the platysma is exposed. Through the incision the hypertrophic platysma portion is resected from the chin just past the hyoid bone. This technique is simpler and more reliable than plication of the medial bands or Z-plasty of the muscle.

Failures are due to irrational expectations of the patient, to certain anatomic factors such as an unfavourably low position of the hyoid bone, exceptionally atrophic skin and subcutaneous tissues, and unaesthetic contours and arches of the facial bony architecture, and to an inadequate surgical technique. Attempts to attain the impossible will always fail.

SURGICAL CORRECTION OF BALDNESS

About 30% of men have androgenetic alopecia and another third are said to have some hair problems (Table 4.1). Surgical correction of

TABLE 4.1   Causes of hair loss and preferential surgical treatment

Type of hair loss	Preferred treatment
Androgenetic alopecia	Punch grafts, alopecia reduction, flaps
Thermal and chemical burns	Surgical excision of scar tissue, punch grafts
Wide scars from trauma	Excision
Burnt-out tinea profunda	Punch grafts
Radiodermatitis	Excision with flap repair and punch grafts for secondary defect
Circumscribed scleroderma, sclerodermie en coup de sabre	Excision, punch grafts
Lichen planus, lupus erythematosus capillitii, necrobiosis, folliculitis decalvans (burnt out)	Punches (single punches may be used and observed for some months before doing a full hair transplant), excision
Postrhytidectomy, traction alopecia	Punch grafts
Loss of eyebrows	Strip grafts

male pattern baldness has therefore become the most frequent cosmetic operation in men[12,13]. A great many articles and books have been written on the surgical treatment of baldness. Different surgical approaches have been proposed[14]:

1. One-stage total excision with primary wound closure from surrounding hair skin – alopecia reduction.
2. One-stage total excision with primary closure of defect with pedicle flap from hairy donor site – scalp flap.
3. Serial excision with gradual decrease of bald area by closure from surrounding hairy skin – serial alopecia reduction.
4. Serial grafting of hair-bearing free autografts from non-alopecia prone hairy skin – punch grafts.
5. One- or multi-step alopecia reduction in combination with free grafts – combined surgical treatment of baldness.

Patient selection

Surgical treatment of bald skin means taking hair from one site and grafting it to the bald spot. Scalp reduction results in a thinning of the skin that is mobilized and stretched for wound closure. To achieve an acceptable result there has to be a reasonable relation of the bald area to the hairy donor area. The donor area must have dense hair. It is wise to see a picture of the patient's father or another relative who is also bald, to judge the fringe of hair that will probably remain.

Contraindications are all diseases with disturbed and delayed wound healing, bleeding disorders, hypertension, mental illness, diabetes mellitus, tendency to hypertrophic scarring and cheloids, scalp infections, immunodeficiencies, and thin hair of a narrow remaining fringe.

The patient must be counselled that several operations will be necessary to obtain a satisfactory result.

Alopecia reduction

Total excision is the treatment of choice for scarring alopecia. It is crucial to avoid too excessive a stretch of the mobilized undermined skin since this will result in a permanent hair loss. The extent of the excision depends on the extent of scarred skin to be removed. Serial excisions may also be necessary for scarring alopecia[14].

Alopecia reduction is usually done under local anaesthesia. Large amounts of 0.5% mepivacaine or lidocaine (lignocaine) with noradrenaline 1:100 000 are injected into the subcutis directly above the galea. The scalp may be trained for some weeks prior to the operation by pinching the scalp skin between the hands, trying to loosen it. This also allows preoperative measurement of the amount of scalp skin to be excised.

The scalp is shampooed with an antiseptic detergent for 2 days before and on the morning of the operation. Photographs are taken prior to the operation. The incision is marked with a waterproof sterile pencil according to the looseness of the skin. The excision may be 10 cm long and up to 4 cm wide in its greatest width.

There are different incision lines. If a multi-stage operation will be

121

necessary the scar of the previous operation should always be removed with the next step. The scalp is sprayed with an antiseptic. The basic incision is crescentic. Since the follicles are very oblique the incision has to be bevelled parallel to the hair shaft to save the roots and the follicles. Usually the incision starts behind the frontal hair line created with punch grafts some weeks previously. It is carried through the galea and the wound edges are elevated with fine hooks to avoid trauma. A blunt curved scissors is inserted between the galea aponeurotica and pericranium, and undermining is obtained by spreading the scissors in the loose connective tissue. After a small area has been undermined further separation of the galea from the pericranium can be most easily performed with the index finger except for the vertex region. This allows an almost bloodless dissection in the parietal area. Clamps are used to compress bleeding vessels of the incision margin until definite haemostasis by ligation or electrocoagulation. Small vessels deep in the wound may be coagulated with the bipolar forceps. After completion of the undermining the medial portion of undermined scalp is pulled over the incision to assess the amount of redundant skin. The excess skin is resected and haemostasis is again obtained with ligation. The mobilized flaps are inelastic since the skin is tightly connected with the underlying galea which is a tough fibrous plate resisting stretching. Advancement can be obtained by multiple galeotomies parallel to the wound edge. Closure of the defect is always achieved in two layers using a running 2/O PDS galea suture and 3/O polypropylene for skin or staples. A running suture is superior if one of the flaps is longer than the other since excess skin length can be evenly distributed with a running suture. Stitches are removed at 12–14 days but it is advantageous to leave them longer if there is no inflammation at the suture marks.

Complications are rare: haematoma, oedema, postoperative pain. Apart from midline excisions which give a scar that often is clearly visible and results in a somewhat unnatural lie of the lateral hair fringe and in a disturbed hair direction in the crown area, Y-, star-, lateral crescent- or J-shaped excisions have been described. The Y-shaped excision allows a larger bald area to be excised and conforms better to the baldness pattern in most patients. Hair direction in the crown is greatly preserved.

After scalp excisions a rewidening of the bald area occurs. This stretch-back may account for one-third to one-half of the immediate postoperative effect in a midline excision. Several scalp reduction operations will invariably thin the skin close to the wound. Particular care has been to be taken for possible later punch grafting in this area[15].

Alopecia reduction by tissue expansion

A subgaleal pocket is made under the scalp skin to be expanded, and an implant that is as long as the bald skin to be replaced is inserted. The incision is made close to the defect to be removed and the galea is divided from the pericranium. This pocket has to be large enough to easily take in the implant. The filling port should be integral with the envelope. Integral valves need no particular dissection for their placement. The incision is closed with non-absorbable sutures in two layers.

Inflation of the implant begins 2 weeks after its implantation and then at weekly intervals. After the desired expansion has been obtained the implant is removed through an incision placed at the border of the bald skin. The incision is prolonged and the expanded skin is pulled over the defect. The area covered by this flap is excised and the expanded scalp is advanced and sutured by two layers into the defect.

Punch grafts

This is the method most widely used and described in detail in numerous books and journal articles[12,13]. Originally devised by Okuda[16] it was popularized by Orentreich 20 years later[17].

Several intrinsic and extrinsic factors determine the outcome of hair transplantation procedures[18]. Intrinsic patient factors are extent of safe donor area and potential bald scalp, hair density per square unit, calibre of individual hair shafts, hair colour, wave or curl of hair, laxity of donor site and bald scalp. Some of these can be improved by surgical alopecia reduction, dyeing and curling of the hair. Extrinsic factors depend on the surgeon and include his skill, talent and his experience, as well as sharpness of the punch, its rotational speed, rapidity of punch advancement, turgor of the donor skin, position of head during harvesting of plugs, haemostasis and oedema prophylaxis, insertion of plugs into recipient site, direction of hair angle at which the hair emerges from the skin, possible suture of plug and pressure bandage after operation[18].

The patient shampoos his hair with an antiseptic detergent the morning before operation. The hair of the donor area, usually the occipital scalp, is trimmed to about 2–3 mm in length. The short hair shafts enable the surgeon to assess the angle at which the shafts emerge from the follicle. The entire scalp is sprayed with an antiseptic. Punches have to be sharpened before each use, and are changed when taking more than 25 plugs.

Even the sharpest punch must not be advanced too fast, in order not to exceed its cutting ability and to avoid distortion of the skin

TABLE 4.2   Donor plugs

Good plug	Poor plug
Quality[18]	
Perfectly cylindrical plug	Cone- or hourglass-shaped plug
No epidermal lipping	Lip of epidermis and papillary dermis
Even, smooth sides	Uneven ragged side
Long axis parallel to hair follicles	Hair follicles not parallel to axis of plug
No hair roots cut, torn or damaged	Hair roots cut, torn or otherwise damaged
Factors influencing the quality of the plug[18]	
Sharp punch	Blunt punch
Internal bevel or angle below 20°	External bevel
Power drive	Hand punch
Slow advancement with minimal pressure	Rapid advancement with pressure
Firm swelling of the donor skin	Soft lax donor skin
Neutral head position	Changing ante- and lateroflexion of patient's head
Dense hair in donor site	Sparse hair in donor site

with splaying of hair follicles. Punch size is usually 4 or 4.5 mm. The punch for the recipient site is 0.5 mm smaller.

Power-driven punches yield better plugs. Optimal rotation speed is 5000 rpm.

Injection of saline to increase the skin's firmness is done immediately before taking the plug. Reinjection of 10 ml or more will be necessary about every 2 minutes. Injection of large amounts of saline also straightens hair follicles and gives a better yield of viable hair follicles in patients with curly hair. To obtain an ideal plug, the patient's head is brought into a neutral position and not turned to the left or right during harvesting (Table 4.2).

Plugs are removed using a fine-toothed forceps. The plug is gently grasped just below the epidermis to avoid crushing of the hair roots, and cut with a small scissors from the attached subcutaneous fat. The portion of the hair root just above the papilla is usually seen as a black dot, and enough fat has to be preserved not to cut the papilla. Using a head magnifier loupe considerably aids in finding the correct plane for trimming away excess subcutaneous fat.

Haemostasis

This is another important point. Suction rodlets dipped into ornipressin solution (POR-8) are inserted into the recipient punch holes until the donor plug is grafted. Pulsating bleeding vessels are electro-coagulated or ligated. Profuse bleeding in the donor area usually stops with skin suture.

Management of the donor area

This varies: the defect is usually sutured in a tongue-and-groove manner. Healing by secondary intention leaves a small round scar shrinking with time.

Plugs are transferred to cold physiological saline and washed to remove hair spicules which would give rise to foreign-body granuloma formation. The plugs are oriented and placed on wet gauze in a sterile Petri dish. Excess fat is trimmed but utmost care has to be taken not to cut the papillae.

Transplantation

This usually starts in the frontal hairline. The frontal hairline is usually shaped as a C, with its convexity facing forward. Temporal recession at both sides make the frontal hairline look more natural. In older patients with a limited donor area a deep recession extended S-shaped hairline may be preferred. Since the plugs retain their hair life-long the hairline must be carefully planned and must not be too deep. The most anterior inch of hair has to be the fullest, and smaller plugs are placed in between larger ones to avoid a scalloped edge. Mini- and micro-grafts further smooth the frontal hairline.

Punches that are 0.5 mm smaller than those for the donor site are used to make the recipient holes. It is wiser to punch the recipient holes as early as possible since haemostasis will then be complete when all donor plugs are ready. Arterial bleeding has to be ligated and since this usually results in considerable distortion of the recipient skin this hole is not filled with a donor plug.

The recipient area may be grafted in three or four sessions in a checkerboard pattern without any grafts touching during each procedure or in full rows. The checkerboard pattern gives overlapping bundles of hairs reducing the appearance of a scalloped edge. The frontal hair has an anterior direction and a rather acute angle of about 30°. The acute angle gives a good overlap of hair shafts and makes a thicker look. The recipient skin is thinner than the donor plugs. Tunnelling of the recipient hole may be necessary. The punch is first inserted vertically, and with further advancement it is gradually tilted until a hole of sufficient depth is created.

The plugs are cautiously grasped with a fine-toothed forceps at the most superficial third of the dermis and gently pushed into the recipient hole. The plug has to lie in the same level as the surrounding skin. This is occasionally difficult to achieve and it is then useful to push the plug deeper into the recipient hole and bring it into the exact level by gently pressing the surrounding skin. Even with tunnelled recipient holes the plugs slide in more easily when held perpendicularly to the scalp. Planting the plugs can be facilitated by using an otic speculum as a funnel. After the plugs have been planted the hair direction of each plug is again checked. Adjustments are made by rotation of the plug. They usually remain in place and need no particular fixing.

A cross-stitch suture technique has several advantages: bleeding is considerably reduced, cobblestone formation is minimized, follicle survival and hair growth are secured and improved, the patient may leave the surgery with only a thin layer of an antibiotic ointment instead of a bandage, the hair may be shampooed at the evening of operation, and physical activity is less restricted. This suture is carried out with 5/O silk or 6/O polypropylene with a firm half-circle needle. Two parallel stitches are made beside the plug and knotted so that the cross comes over the centre of the plug. This suture technique is particularly useful where the recipient skin is much thinner than the donor plug and for atrophic scars[19]. Usually not more than 80 plugs are transplanted per session.

Mini- and micrografts

These have further improved the creation of a natural-looking hairline. A simple technique uses plugs with hair follicles directly on their periphery. The plug is held at its epidermal margin with a fine forceps and superficial incisions are made with a No. 11 blade on the sides of the potential micrograft. The blades of a fine sharp scissors are placed into these notches. While pressing the scissors downward upon the plug, the micrograft between the scissor blades is slightly elevated and can be cut beginning at the epidermis and proceeding to the papillae. The micrografts are inserted 1–3 mm anterior to the hairline created with standard grafts.

The recipient hole is produced with a large-bore injection needle which is appropriately angled, pushed through the skin and left in place for 30–60 seconds. This time span is sufficient to retain the circular tunnel shape for the few moments that are necessary to insert the micrograft. When it is implanted its epidermal surface is trimmed away and the entire graft is pushed just below the level of the surrounding epidermis. When the skin closes in, the micrograft is completely buried. After about 3 months the hair pierces through the epidermis covering the invisible micrograft. Scarring is virtually non-existent.

Complications

Complications are rare in cases operated by experienced surgeons.

Combined treatment of androgenetic alopecia

Since alopecia reduction alone is applicable only to patients who have balding of the crown with an intact frontal hairline, and since Hamilton types IV to VI may not have enough donor area left to cover the bald area, a combination of punch grafts and alopecia reduction may be used[20]. Most commonly the frontal hairline is first created using punch grafts. The bald vertex and midscalp are then reduced by serial excision. When planning a combination of punch grafts and alopccia rcductions it is wisc to takc into considcration the fact that the frontal hairline will recede in its lateral parts, thus deepening the temporal recession. Scalp reductions are recommended to be performed only 6 weeks after the frontal hairline has been established; 6–10 weeks should elapse between serial scalp reductions[20].

Flaps

Due to the refinements in punch grafting and alopecia reduction techniques, flaps will probably become less often used. There are different types of flaps that may be used such as rotation, transposition, and island artery flaps. However, the flap most widely used is the Juri transposition flap that has been slightly modified by several authors.

Implantation of synthetic hair fibres

The implantation of artificial hair fibres (Table 4.3) was criticized because of serious complications. A material that seems to be much better tolerated is now available – Nido hair with fibres made of polyethylene terephthalate[21].

TABLE 4.3 Synthetic hair and hair transplantation

Synthetic hair	Hair transplantation
Advantages:	Disadvantages:
Unlimited amount of fibres available	Limited amount of transplants
Single hair implantation	Transplantation of hair bushes
Fibre removal without scar	Operation is definite and irretrievable
Immediate postoperative result	Result only after 6 months to 1 year
One or two implantations sufficient	Usually three or four sessions, or more
Disadvantages:	Advantages:
Risk of postoperative infection	Usually no infection
Gradual loss of hair requires new implantations	No hair loss
Feeling of artificial synthetic material	Natural hair
Consistent medical control required	
Formation of peri-'pilar' pits	
Special hair stylist required	
Consistent particular care necessary	

LIPOSUCTION

Indications

Indications for liposuction are localized fat deposits on lower abdomen, hips, buttocks, flanks, around the knees and ankles, beneath the chin, from the jowls and nasolabial folds, large lipomas, pseudogynaecomastia, buffalo humps, and puffed sleeve deformity in Launois–Bensaude syndrome. Generalized obesity cannot be treated with liposuction[22].

129

Patient selection

This is often more difficult than is anticipated. Preoperative and postoperative photographs are essential. Marking of the fat deposits is always done in a standing position in a relaxed state and with the muscles contracted. The fat deposit to be removed is encircled and any area with less fat gets an extra mark to be spared. The periphery of the deposit is marked with a broken line. The incisions are drawn, usually hardly larger than the diameter of the suction cannula and in a hidden place. At least two, sometimes even multiple, incisions are performed wherever possible. The tunnels to be created may be marked, too, preferably with another colour, and a criss-cross pattern is drawn. The main direction of the tunnels is vertical, since horizontal suction tunnels would result in, or increase, waving and furrowing. The ideal candidate is a young slender person with a well-circumscribed fat deposit and a tight skin. Truncal and extremity liposuction surgery is usually done under *general anaesthesia*.

Surgical technique

This involves incisions at the margin of the fat deposit. The correct suction plane is found by spreading scissors perpendicular to the plane just above the fascia; it should be at least 1–2 cm below the dermis to avoid waving. The skin and subcutaneous fat is grasped with the left hand and lifted. A blunt solid tapered tunnelling instrument is inserted through the incision and pushed to the centre of the fat which is controlled with the left hand while creating new radial tunnels in the form of spokes of a wheel. The same procedure is done from another incision opposite the first one to form a latticework of tunnels. The suction cannula is then inserted into the tunnels with its opening face downward. The fat is suctioned from the depths of the tunnels. A uniform layer of fat has to remain between dermis and tunnels. No fan-like motion must be performed with the cannula. The cannula is rapidly moved forward and backward, approximately ten to fifteen times per tunnel with every fifth motion going beyond the circular mark to the periphery with the broken line. A flow of pure yellow fat should be seen through the clear suction tube.

After about 15 strokes blood can be seen in the tube. The cannula is withdrawn and entered into the next tunnel. With more and more fat being removed the left hand that formerly had grasped the skin and adipose tissue is opened and used to press and push the cannula down and guide it to the depths of the tunnels. When the satisfactory contour has been reached the tunneller is again reinserted into the tunnels and extended into the non-treated surrounding adipose tissue in order to get a smoother transition from the periphery to the former fat accumulation. The fat is also mobilized by massaging motions of the surgeon's left hand during this procedure.

At least two round suction drains are placed into the wound. Closed suction drainage is maintained for 2–3 days.

A tight tape garment with elastic tape is applied for 8 days. The pressure of the tape is to collapse the tunnels in the adipose tissue, control bleeding and support the skin. Care has to be taken to avoid any folds. After removal of the tape the patient has to wear a tight-fitting above-the-knee hose and a long-legged elastic panty-girdle for another 3 weeks. After 1 month the patient is to start vigorous massage over all suctioned areas. Particularly in patients over 35 years of age there may be redundant skin after liposuction. Scarring and shrinking of newly formed connective tissue in the subcutis may reduce this excess of skin by up to 30%.

Liposuction probably results in a permanent removal of the fat pads since no new fat cells are produced even when the patient gains weight.

Complications

Complications are pain and soreness, but haemorrhage is rare. Numbness is due to nerve injury but usually fades. Irregular contours with depressions, dimples or furrows may occur but often smooth out to some degree. In general, improvement only comes some weeks after liposuction.

Equipment

Different items of equipment are now available. The suction machine has to build up a negative pressure of 1 atmosphere. It is recommended to use it with two suction bottles, which makes it easier to control the amount of fat and fluid suctioned from symmetrical locations. The tubing is transparent and may be reinforced. Blunt solid tapered bullet-shaped tunnellers are now used to make the tunnels before the actual suction procedure, though this may also be accomplished using the cannula without suction. Cannulae are short or long and have diameters from 2 to 10 mm. They are straight or gently curved. Most have one opening, but the thinner ones may have three or even five apertures. The aperture edges have to be blunt to avoid cutting or curettage. Cannulae for facial liposuction are flat.

References

1. Braun-Falco, O., De Dulanto, F., Epstein, E., Bernstein, G. and Hanke, C. W. (1985). A decade of dermatologic surgery. *J. Dermatol. Surg. Oncol.*, **11**, 199–205
2. Stegman, S. J. and Tromovitch, T. (1984). *Cosmetic Dermatologic Surgery.* (Chicago and London: Year Book Medical Publishers)
3. Haneke, E. (1984). Indikationsabwägung bei der operativen Therapie benigner Hautveränderungen. In Konz, B. and Braun-Falco, O. (eds.) *Komplikationen in der operativen Dermatologie.* pp. 141–6. (Berlin, Heidelberg, New York and Tokyo: Springer)
4. Petres, J. (1985). Therapie des Rhinophyms. *Hautarzt*, **36**, 433–5
5. Staindl, O. (1985). Indications of the fibrin sealant in facial plastic surgery. *Facial Plast. Surg.*, **2**, 323–9
6. Zoltan, J. (1977). *Atlas der chirurgischen Schnitt- und Nahttechnik zur Erzielung optimaler Wundheilung.* (Basel, München, Paris, London, New York and Sydney: S. Karger)
7. Haneke, E. (1981). The immediate removal of accidental tattoos. In Bernstein, L. (ed.) *Aesthetic Surgery.* Vol. 1, pp. 189–90. (New York: Grune & Stratton)
8. Haneke, E. (1977). Möglichkeiten und Grenzen der kombinierten Spalthautlappen- und Schleiftherapie von Tätowierungen. *Hautarzt*, **28**, Suppl. II, 60–1
9. Landes, E. (1985). Dermabrasion und ihre Problematik. *Z. Hautkr.*, **60**, 1337–49
10. Roenigk, H. H. jr. (1985). Dermabrasion: state of the art. *J. Dermatol. Surg. Oncol.*, **11**, 306–14

11. Resnik, S. S. (1984). Chemical peeling with trichloroacetic acid. *J. Dermatol. Surg. Oncol.*, **10**, 550
12. Unger, W. P. (1978). *Hair Transplantation.* (New York: Marcel Dekker)
13. Norwood, O. T. and Shiell, R. C. (eds.) (1984). *Hair Transplant Surgery.* 2nd Edn. (Springfield/III: C. C. Thomas)
14. Friederich, H. C. (1970). Indikation und Technik der operativ-plastischen Behandlung des Haarverlustes. *Hautarzt*, **21**, 197-202
15. Nordström, R. E. A. (1984). Scalp kinetics in multiple excisions for correction of male pattern baldness. *J. Dermatol. Surg. Oncol.*, **10**, 991-5
16. Okuda, S. (1939). Klinische und experimentelle Untersuchungen über die Transplantation von lebenden Haaren. *Jpn. J. Dermatol. Urol.*, **46**, 135-8
17. Orentreich, N. (1959). Autografts in alopecias and other selected dermatological conditions. *Ann. NY Acad. Sci.*, **83**, 463-79
18. Alt, H. (1984). Evaluation of donor harvesting techniques in hair transplantation. *J. Dermatol. Surg. Oncol.*, **10**, 799-806
19. Orentreich, N. and Orentreich, D. S. (1984). 'Cross stitch' suture technique for hair transplantation. *J. Dermatol. Surg. Oncol.*, **10**, 970-1
20. Roenigk, H. H. (1985). Combined surgical treatment of male pattern alopecia. *Cutis*, **35**, 570-7
21. Taniguchi, S. (1984). A histopathological study of the percutaneous implantation of polyester fibers. *Aesth. Plast. Surg.*, **8**, 67-74
22. Dolsky, R. L. (1984). Body sculpturing by lipo-suction extraction. *Aesth. Plast. Surg.*, **8**, 75-83

INDEX